I Am Healthy!

Affirmations for Health and Well-Being

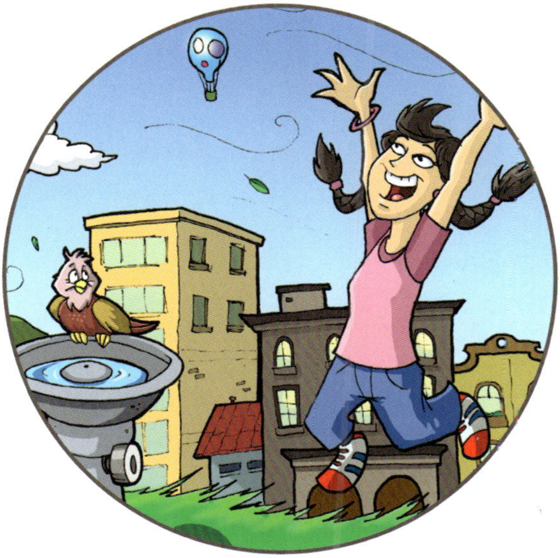

by Steve Viglione

Creative Director, Dr. Marilyn Powers
Illustrated by Mauricio Hoffman
Spanish Translation by Julietta Ingham
Graphic Design by (in)Spire Graphics
Healthy Scoop pages by Vicki Whiting of Kid Scoop®
Edited by Vicki Worthington

English-Spanish Edition

Published by The I AM Foundation
www.iamfoundation.org

Follow us on f

FSC www.fsc.org MIX Paper from responsible sources FSC® C008955

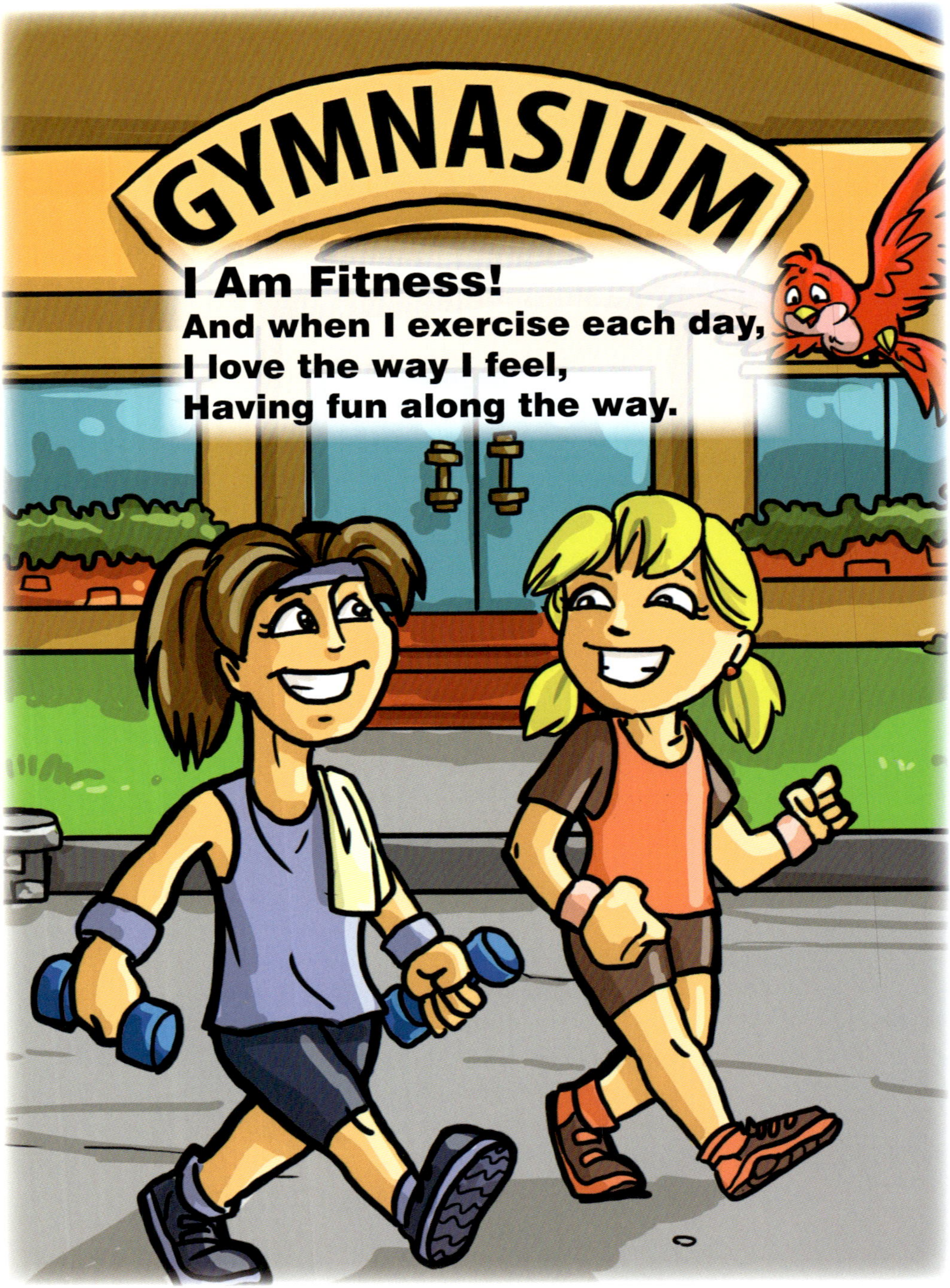

I Am Fitness!
And when I exercise each day,
I love the way I feel,
Having fun along the way.

Yo Soy y estoy en buen estado físico!
Y cuando me ejercito cada día,
me encanta cómo me siento.
Y esa alegría guía mi camino.

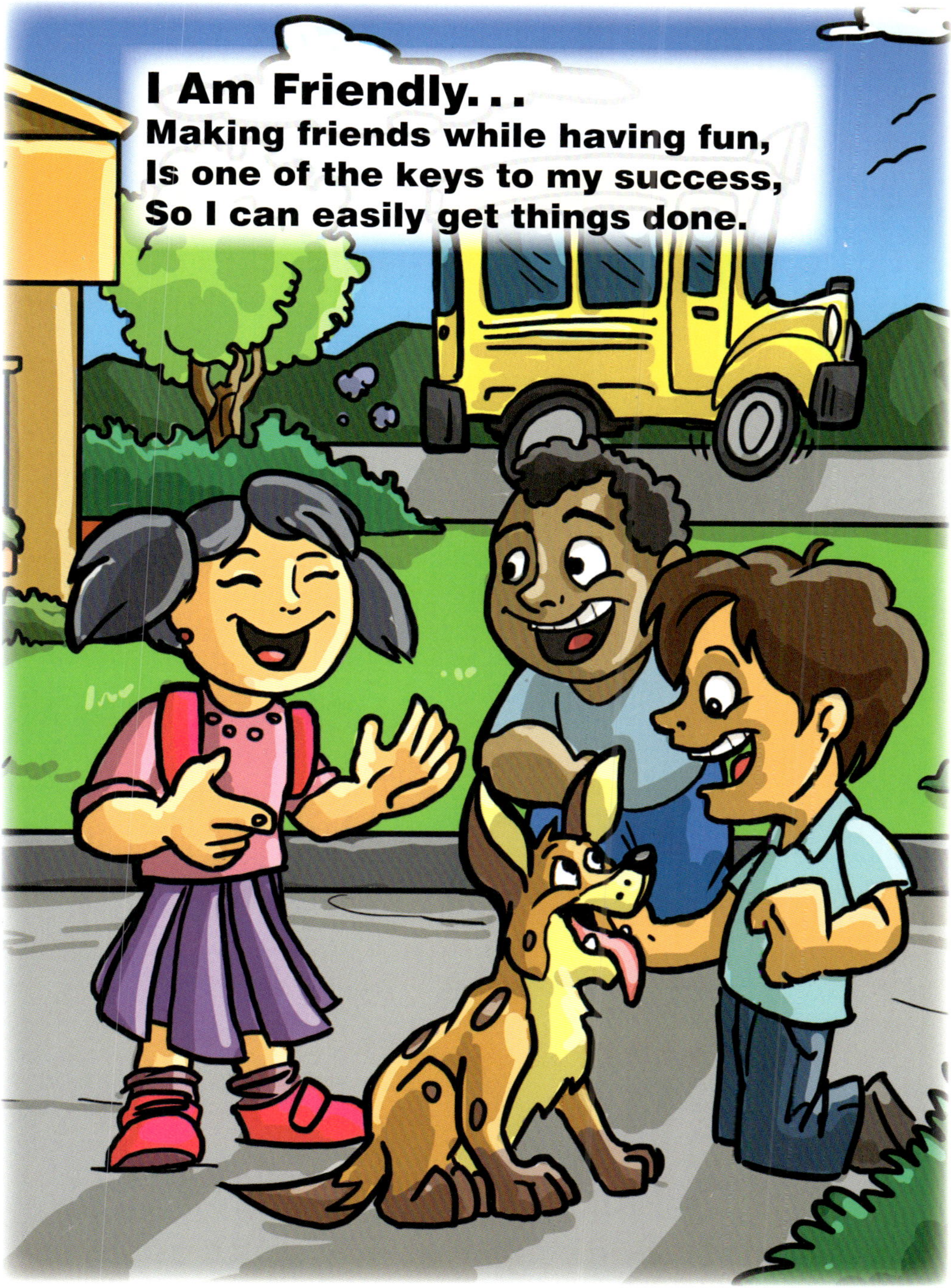

Yo Soy Amigable...

Haciendo amigos mientras me divierto,
es una de las claves de mi éxito,
para terminar de hacer las cosas fácilmente.

I Am Active!

And I love to exercise my heart,
Because when I run, walk, or swim,
My health soars off the chart!

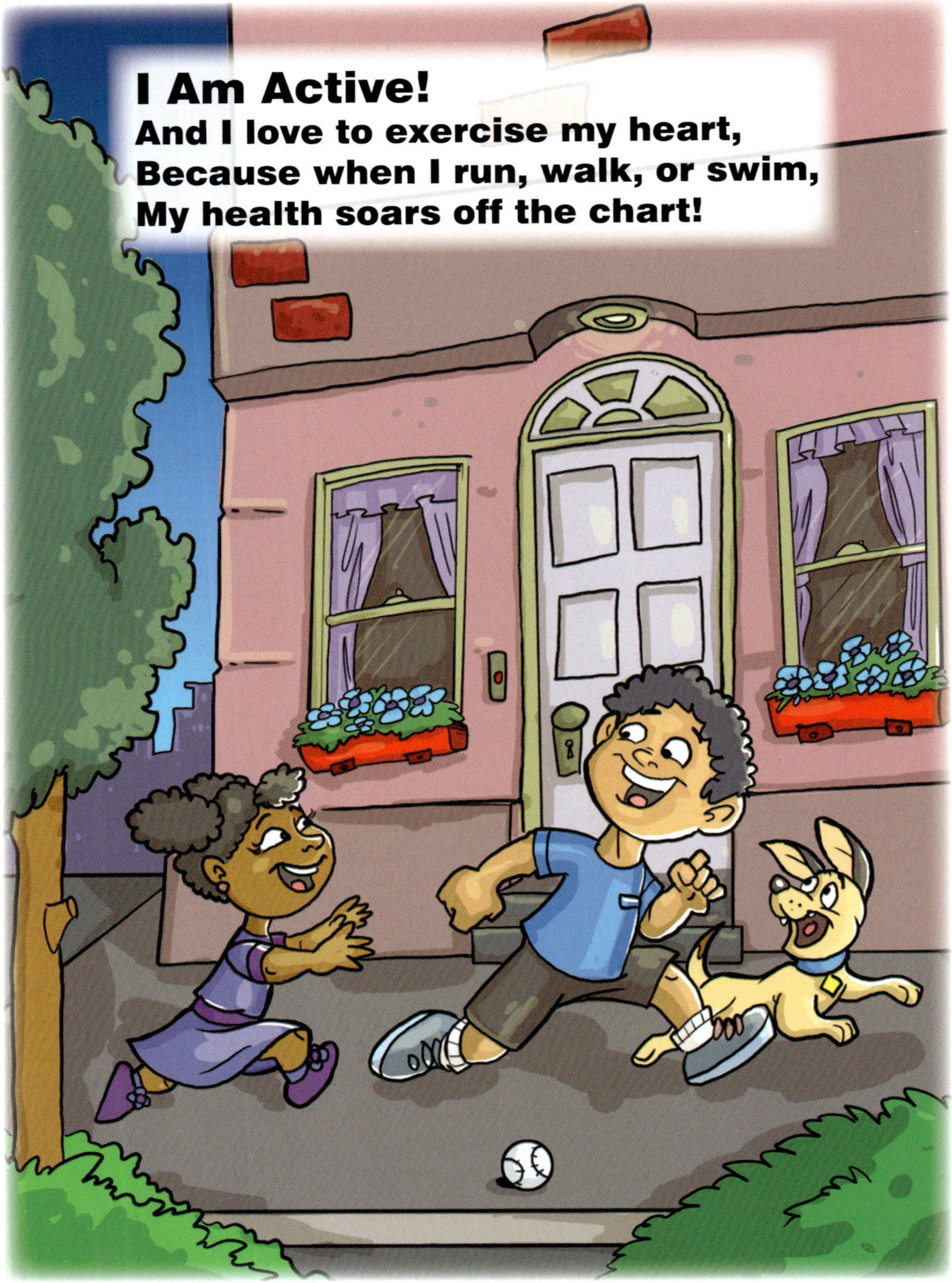

Yo Soy Activo!

Me encanta ejercitar mi corazón.
Cuando corro, nado, o paseo,
mi salud es fuera de serie!

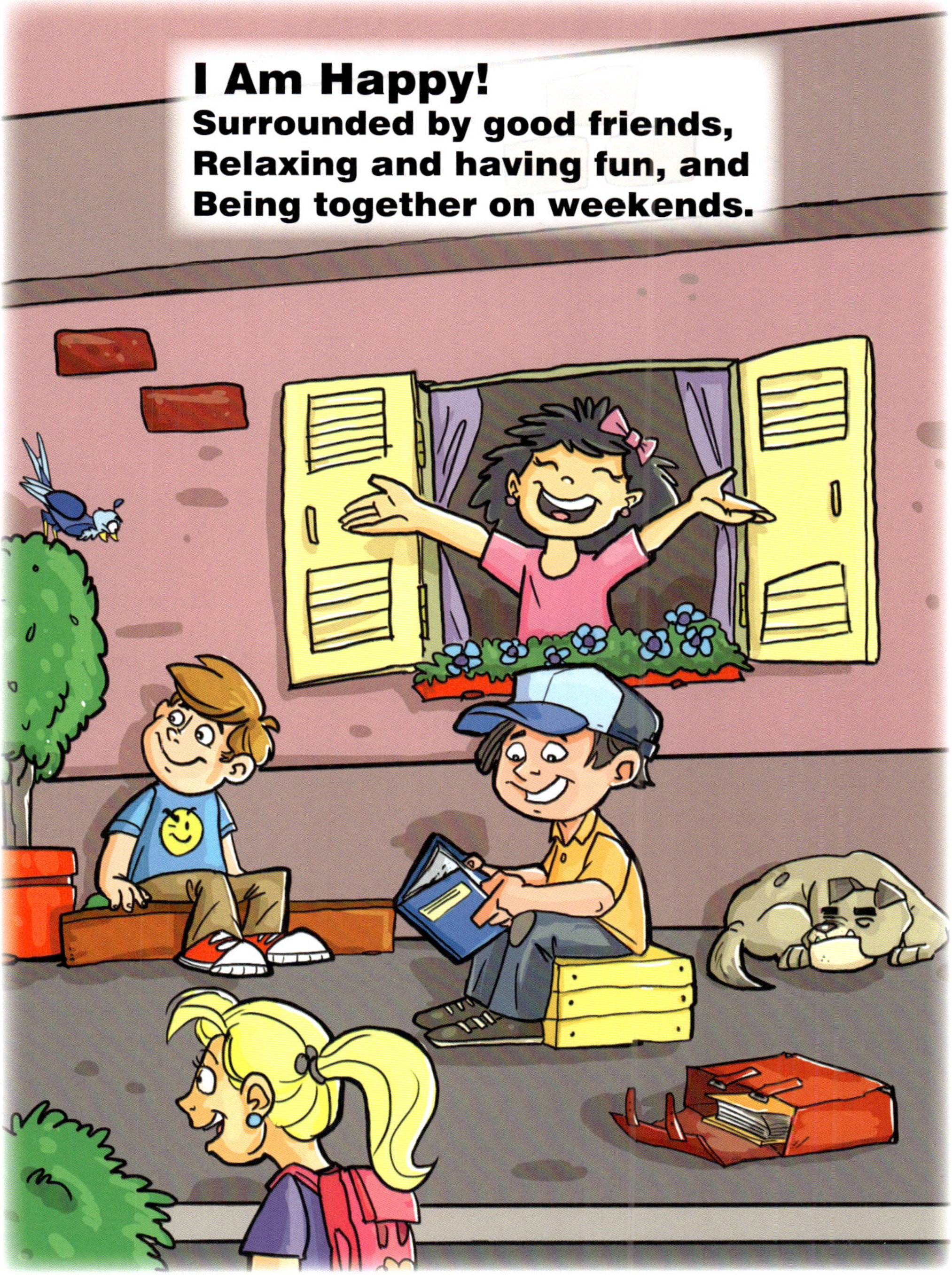

Yo Soy Feliz!

Y rodeado de buenos amigos.
Me relajo y me divierto,
junto con ellos los fines de semana.

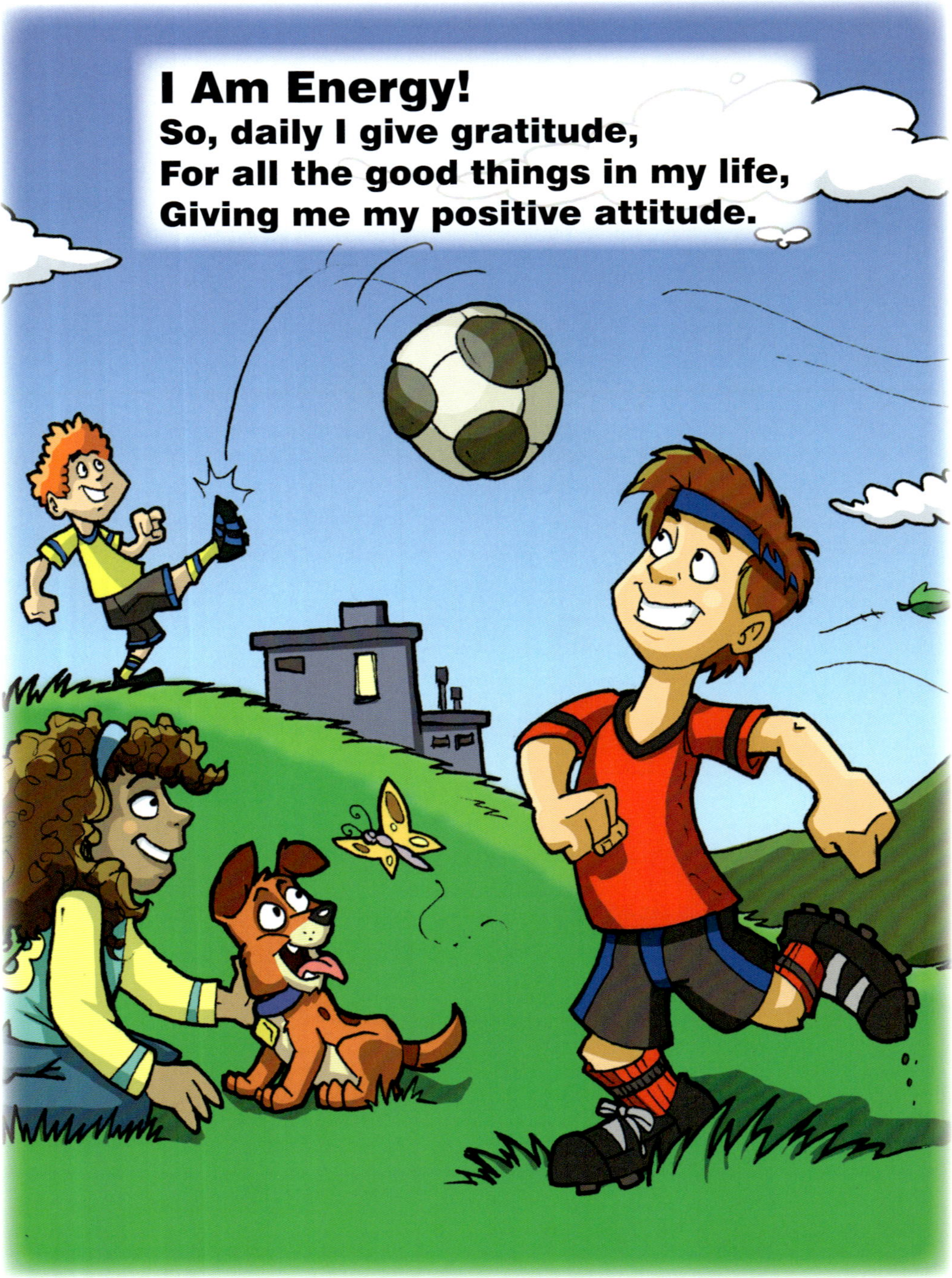
I Am Energy!
So, daily I give gratitude,
For all the good things in my life,
Giving me my positive attitude.

Yo Soy Energía!

**Diariamente doy gracias por todas
las cosas buenas en mi vida.
Y me doy a mí mismo una actitud positiva.**

I Am Joyful!

So I jump for joy,
And when I play outside,
It’s like enjoying my favorite toy.

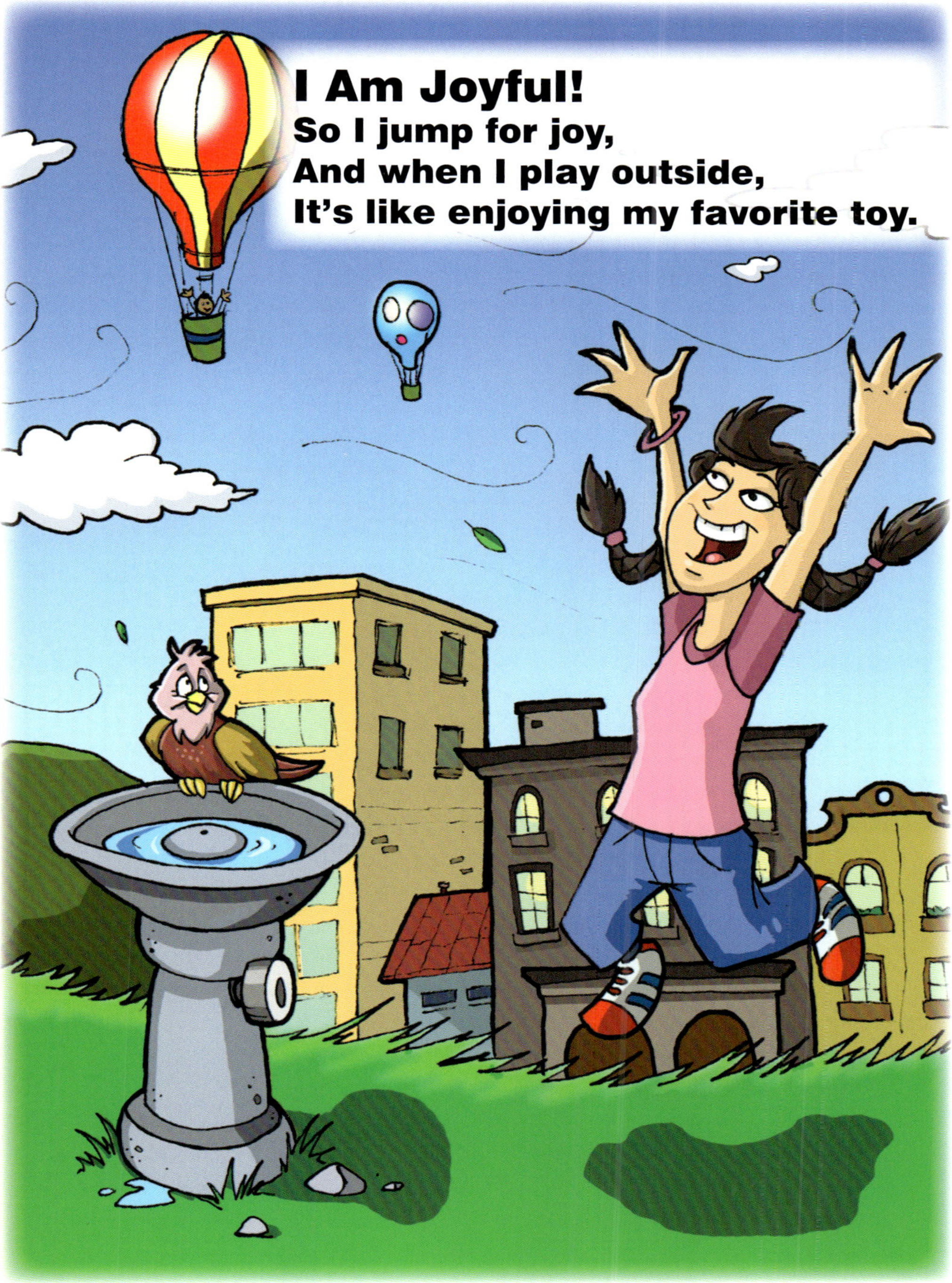

Yo Soy Alegre!

Por lo tanto brinco de alegría,
y cuando salgo a jugar afuera,
es como si disfrutara mi juguete favorito.

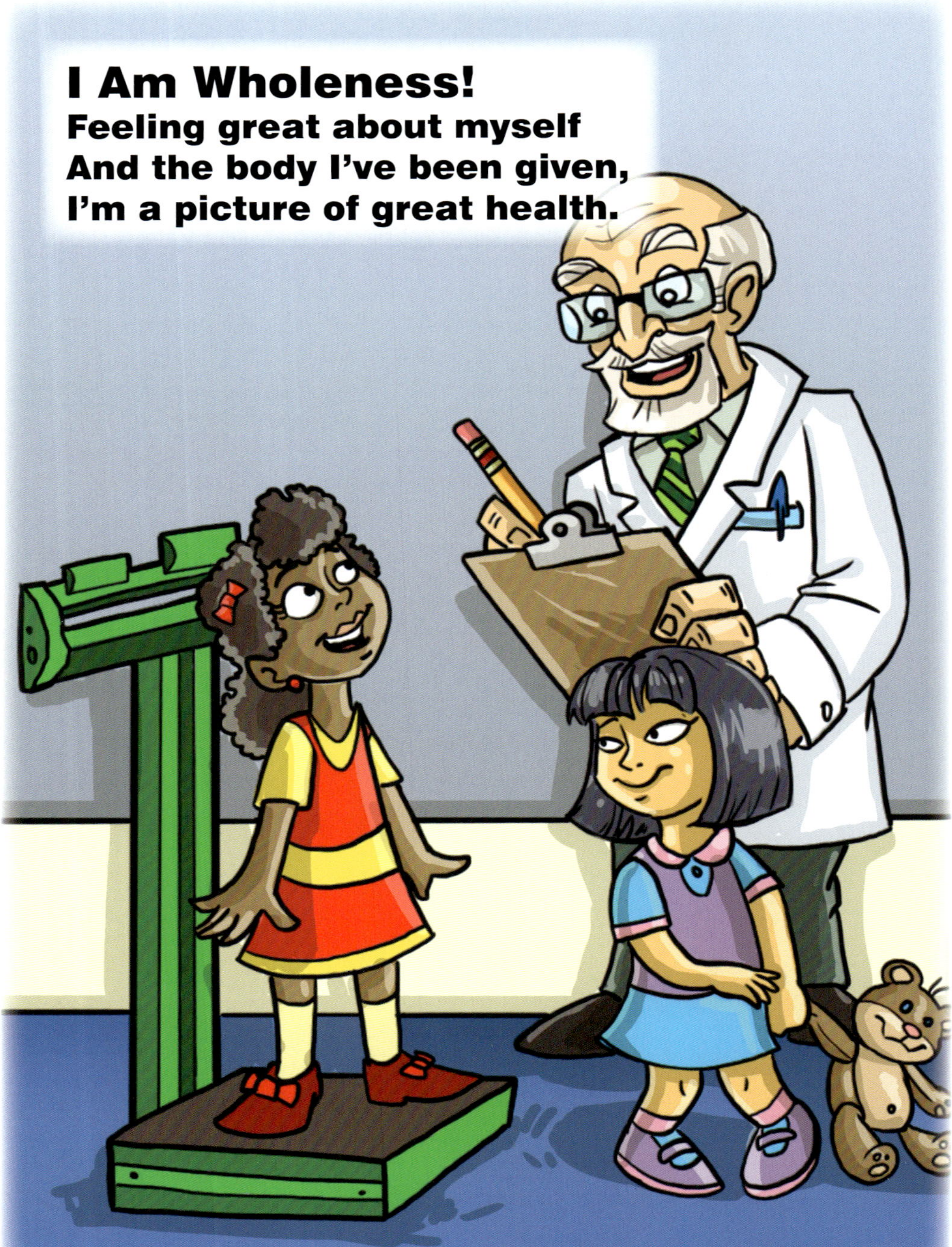
I Am Wholeness!
Feeling great about myself
And the body I've been given,
I'm a picture of great health.

Yo Soy Plenitud!

Sintiéndome bien conmigo mismo
y con el cuerpo que se me ha dado.
Soy la viva imagen de la salud.

I Am Consistent!

**Going to the dentist or the doc,
Getting regular check-ups,
So my health runs like a clock.**

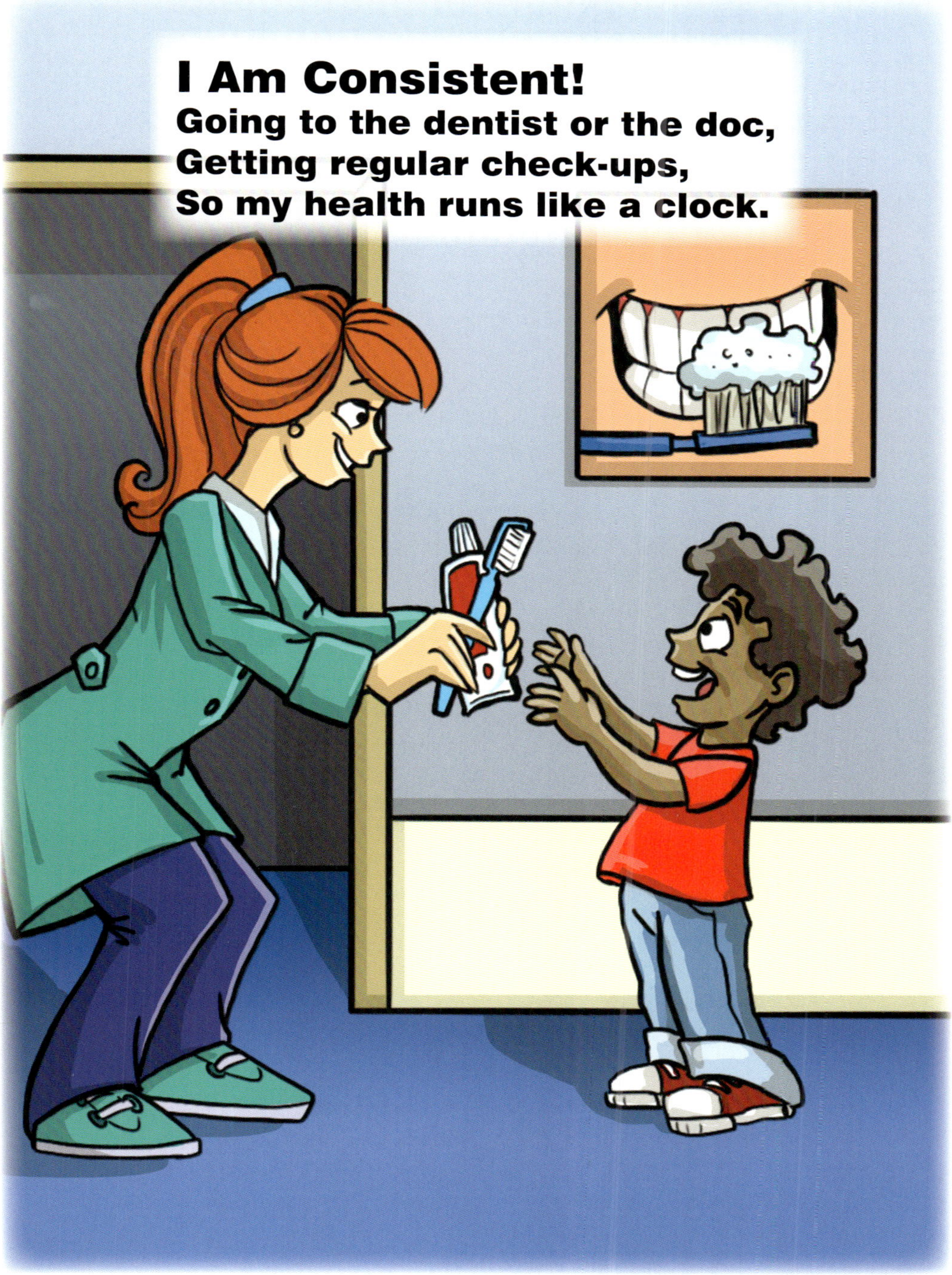

Yo Soy Consistente!

**Cuando visito al dentista o al doctor,
y me checo regularmente,
mi salud funciona como un reloj.**

I Am Wise!

I make good choices each and every day,
Which support my health and well-being.
Now, I'm on my way.

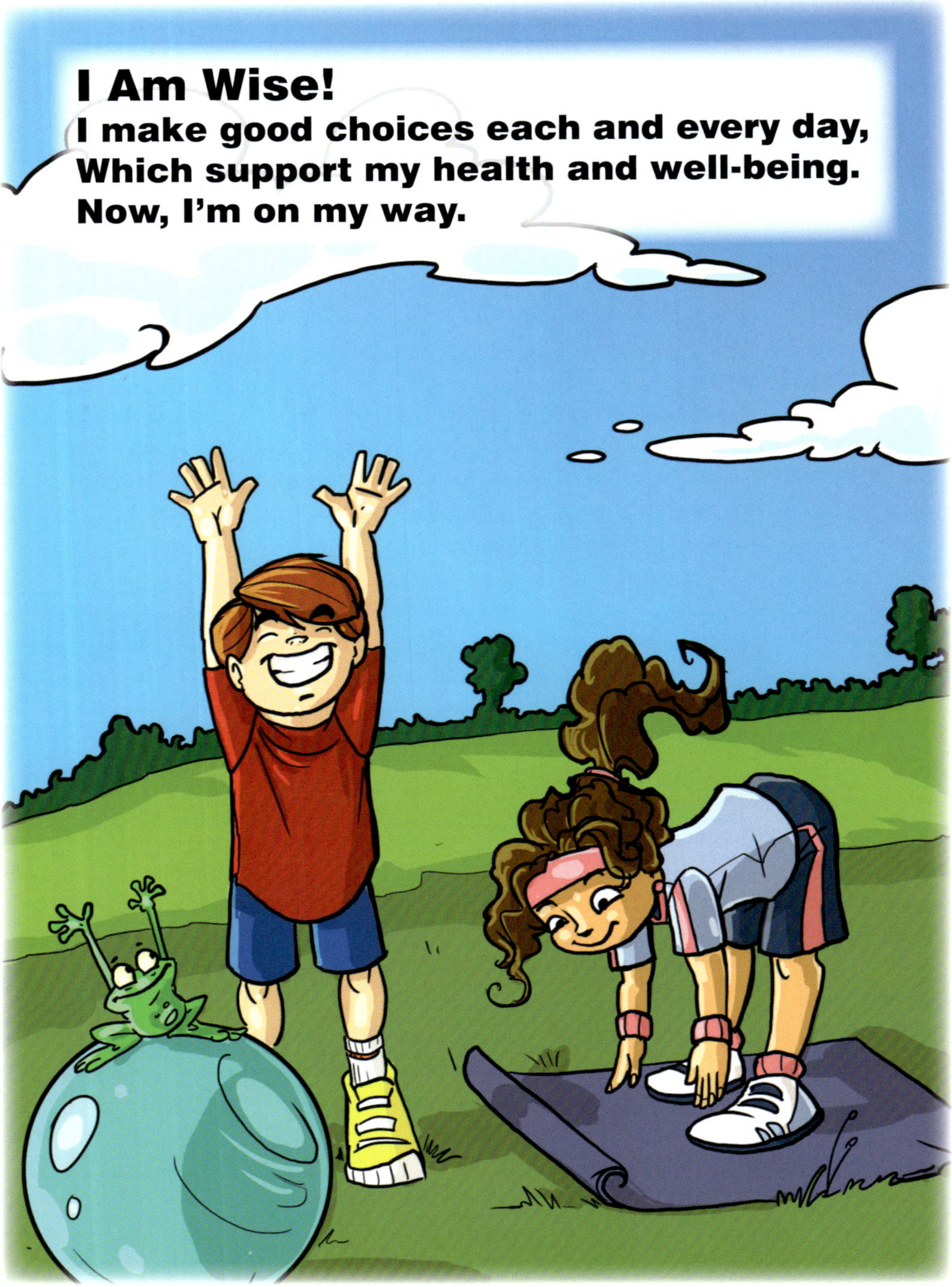

Yo soy Sabio!

Y tomo buenas decisiones cada día,
y todos los días que apoyan mi salud y bienestar.
Ahora sé el camino a seguir.

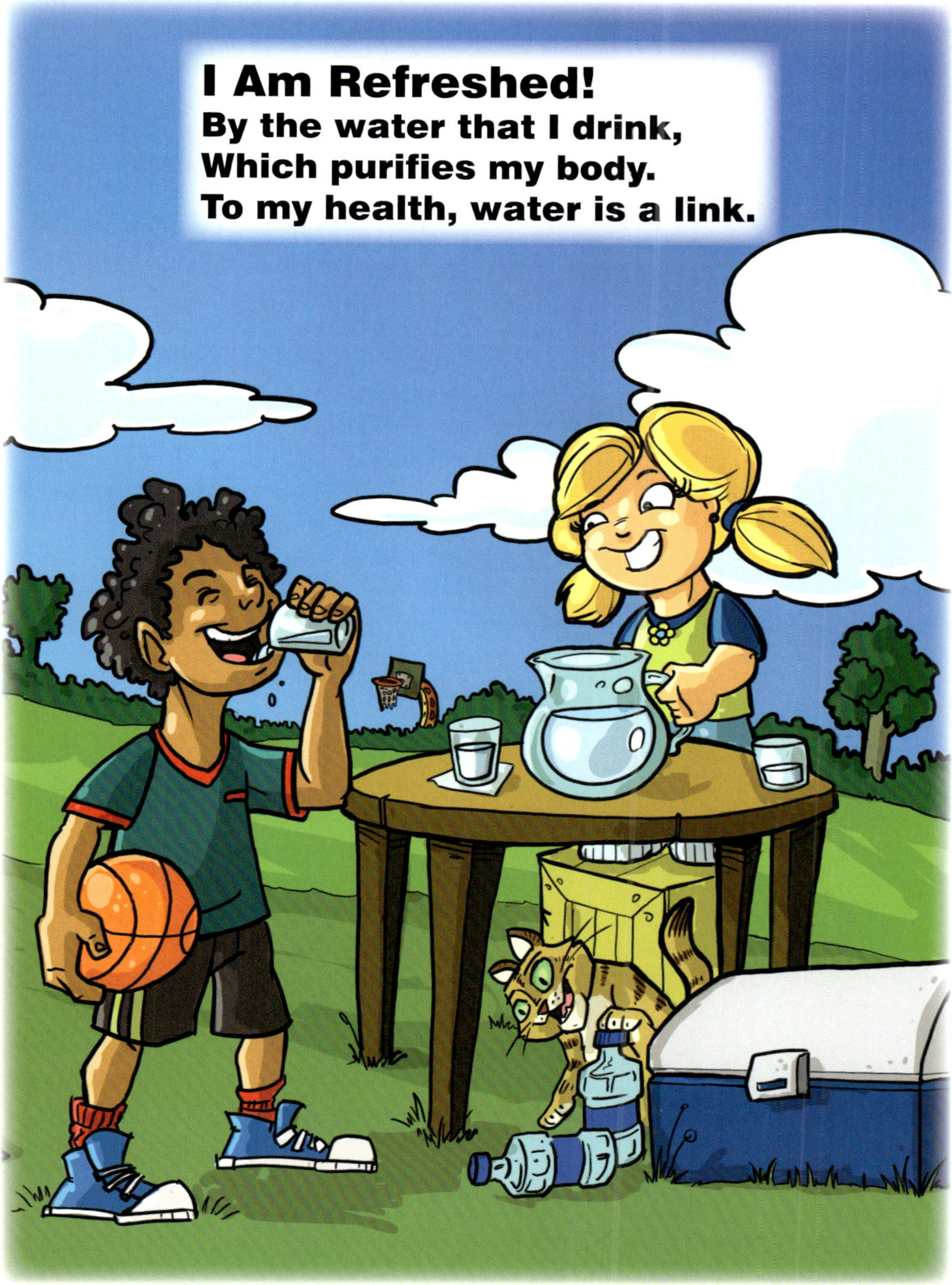
I Am Refreshed!
By the water that I drink,
Which purifies my body.
To my health, water is a link.

Yo Soy y me siento fresco!
Por que el agua que tomo,
purifica mi cuerpo.
El agua es el enlace para mi salud.

I Am Nature . . .

And I love to hike and walk
To see the sights and hear the sounds
From maybe a wise, old owl or a hawk.

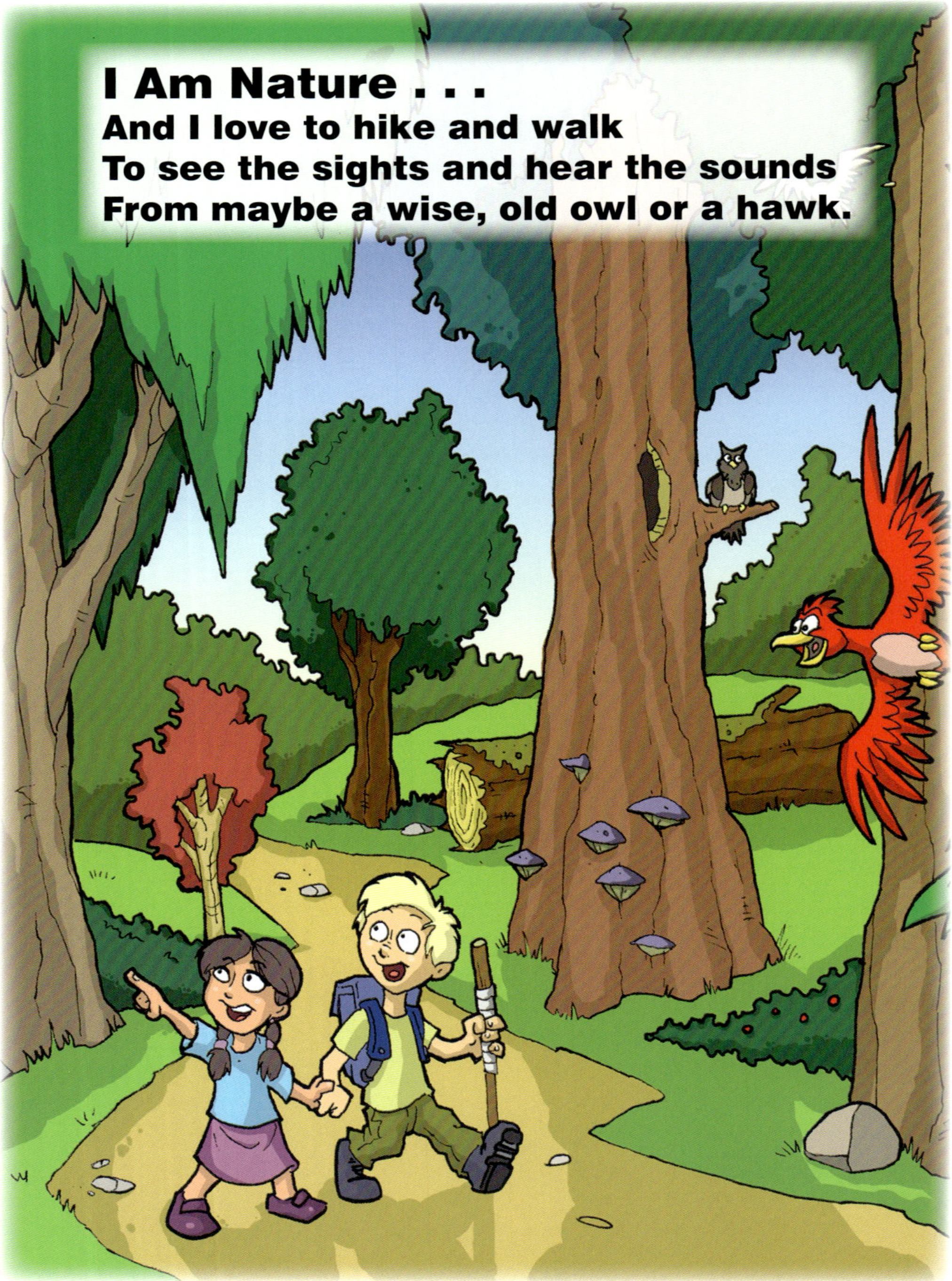

Yo soy Naturaleza . . .

Me encanta ir de excursión y caminar.
Ver los lugares de interés y escuchar los sonidos,
tal vez de un búho viejo y sabio, o de un halcón.

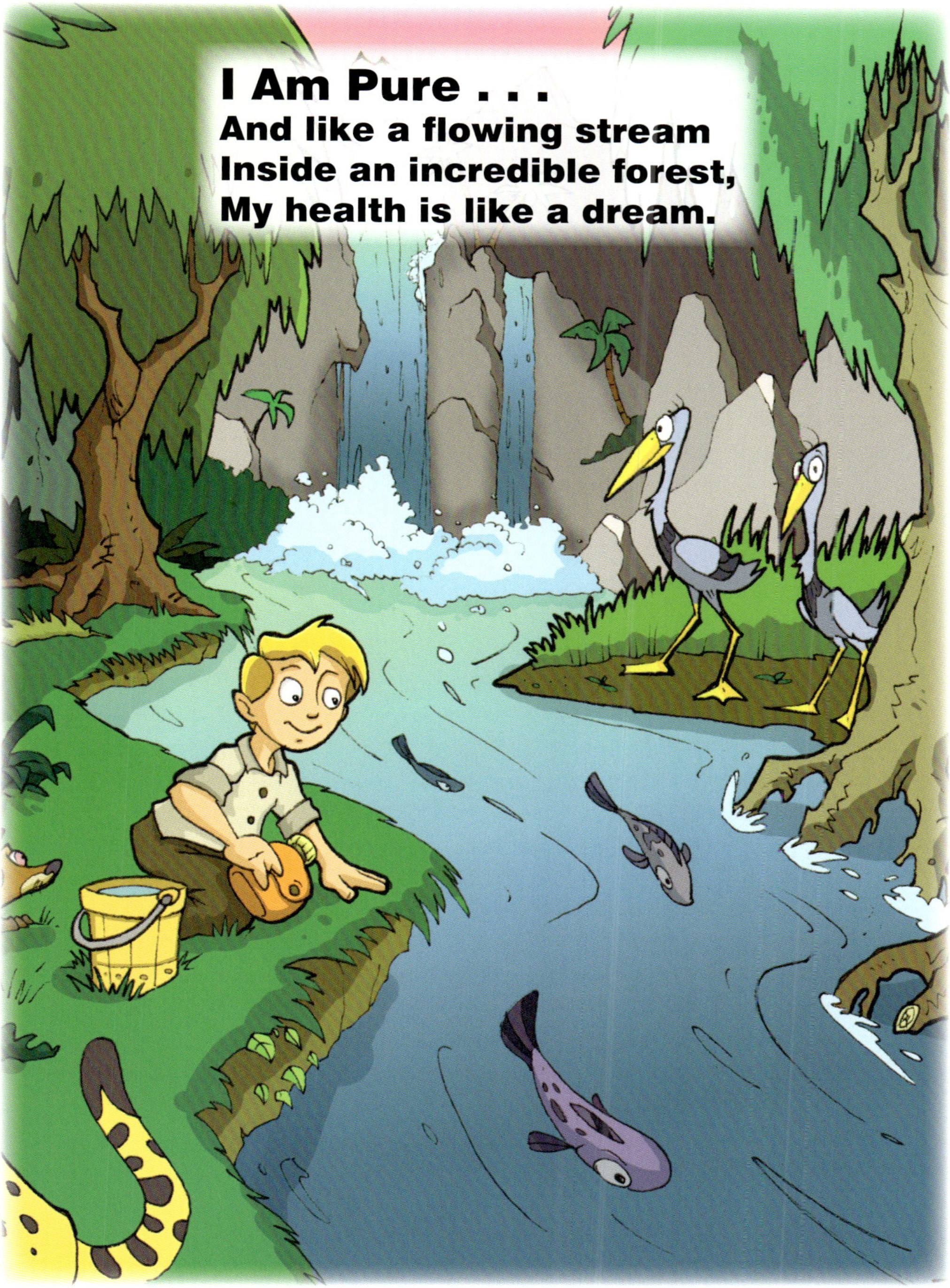
I Am Pure . . .
And like a flowing stream
Inside an incredible forest,
My health is like a dream.

Yo Soy Puro...

Como la corriente que fluye
dentro de un bosque increíble.
Mi salud es como un sueño.

I Am All Natural . . .
And I create a healthy me.
Choosing nature's snacks and treats,
Like an apple from a tree!

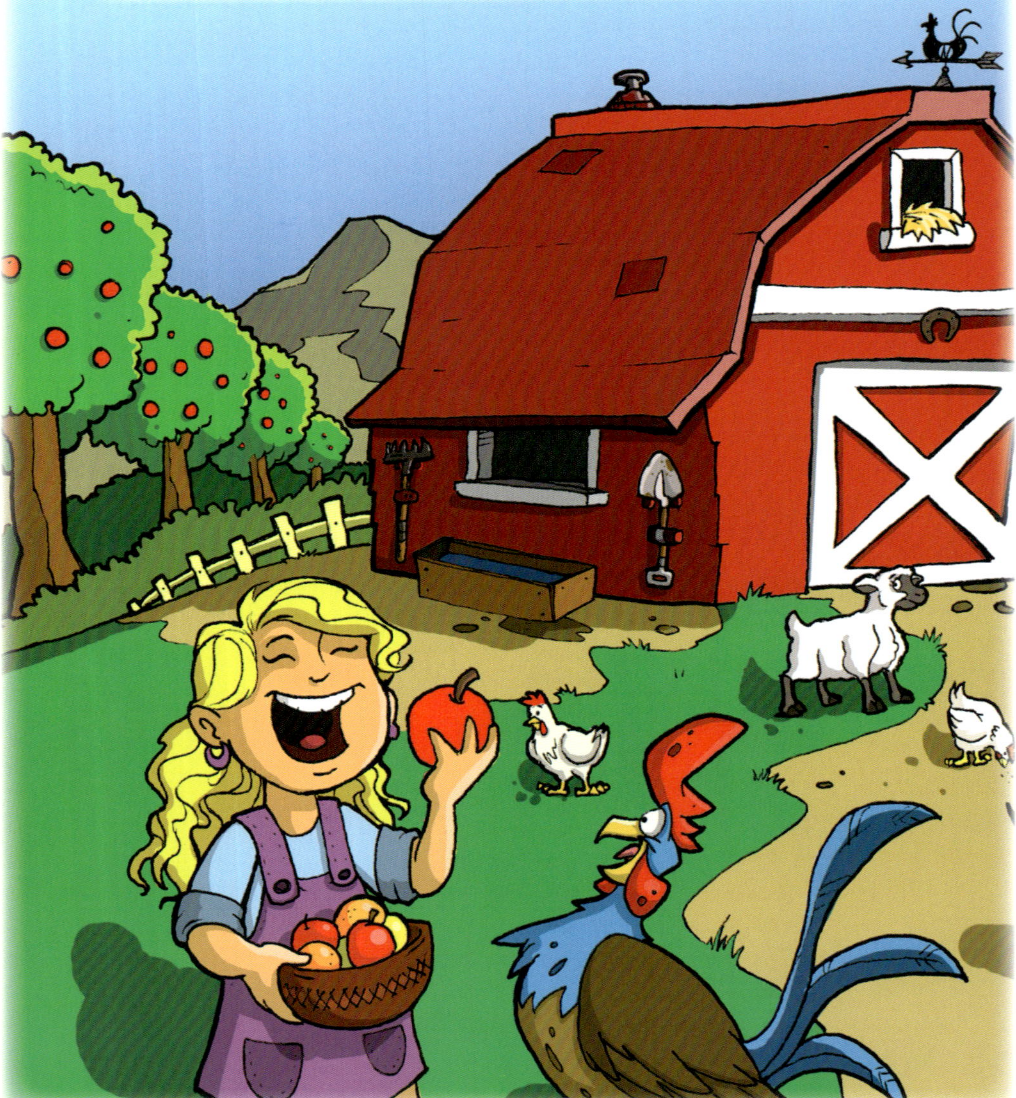

Yo Soy Todo Natural. . .
Y he creado un Yo sano.
Elijo de la naturaleza mis antojos y bocadillos,
como la manzana de un árbol!

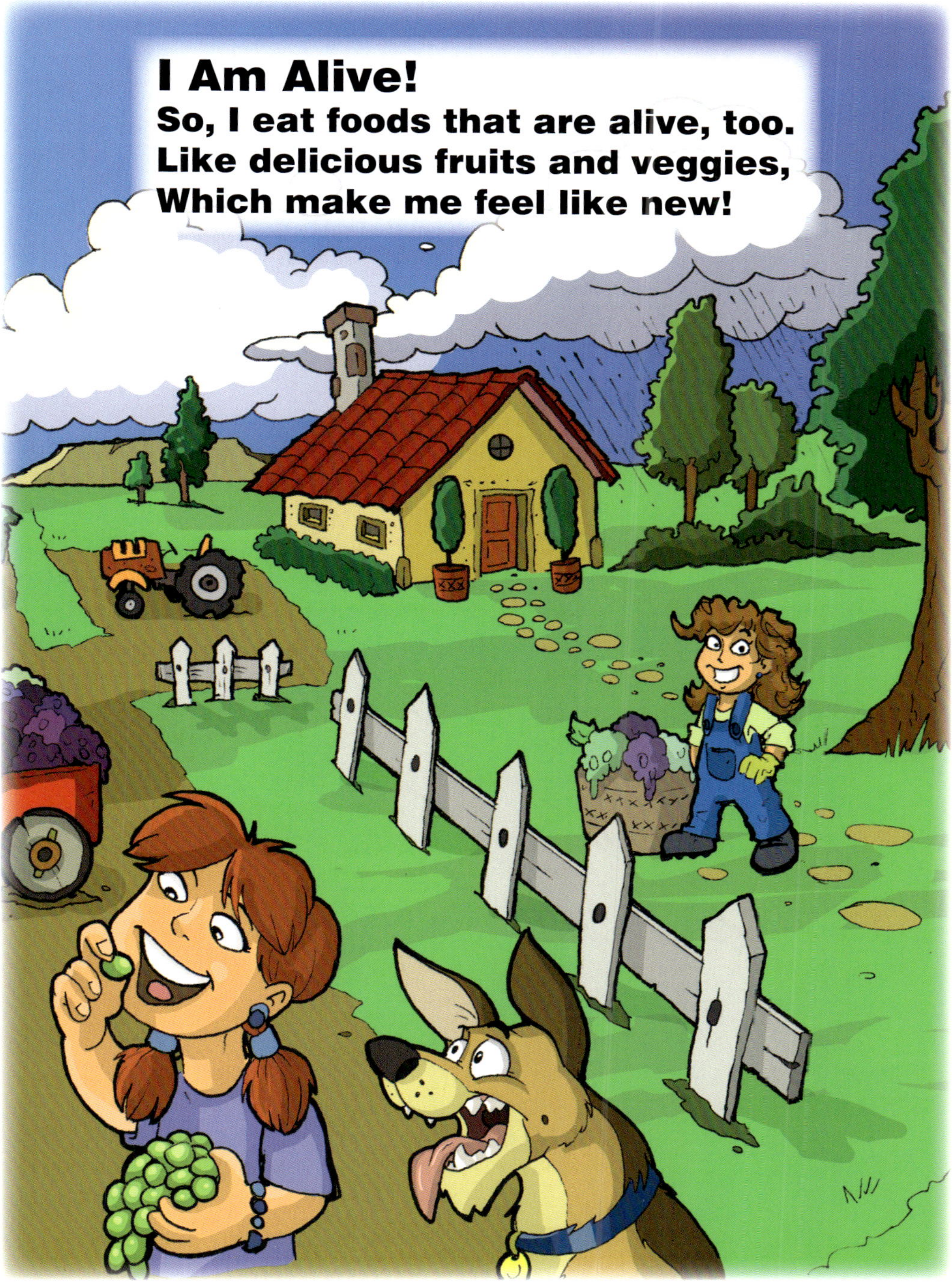
I Am Alive!
So, I eat foods that are alive, too.
Like delicious fruits and veggies,
Which make me feel like new!

Yo estoy Vivo!

Así que como alimentos vivos,
también como deliciosas frutas y vegetales.
Los cuales me hacen sentir como nuevo!

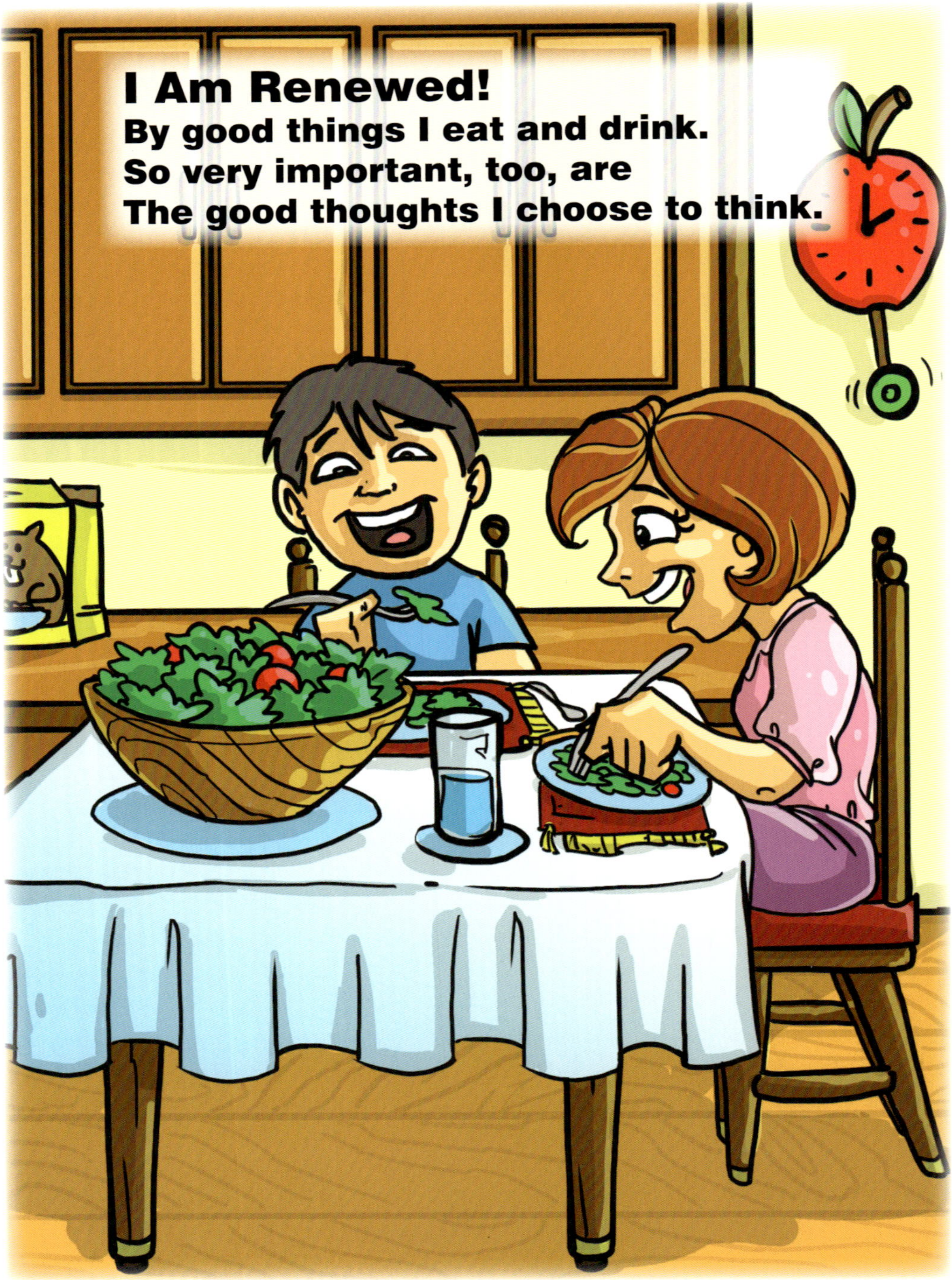
I Am Renewed!
By good things I eat and drink.
So very important, too, are
The good thoughts I choose to think.

Yo Soy y me renuevo!

Por que las cosas buenas que como y bebo son tan importantes también, como los buenos pensamientos que elijo pensar.

I Am a Reader . . .

**I read to learn what's good for me.
When it comes to good nutrition,
I take action! That's the key!**

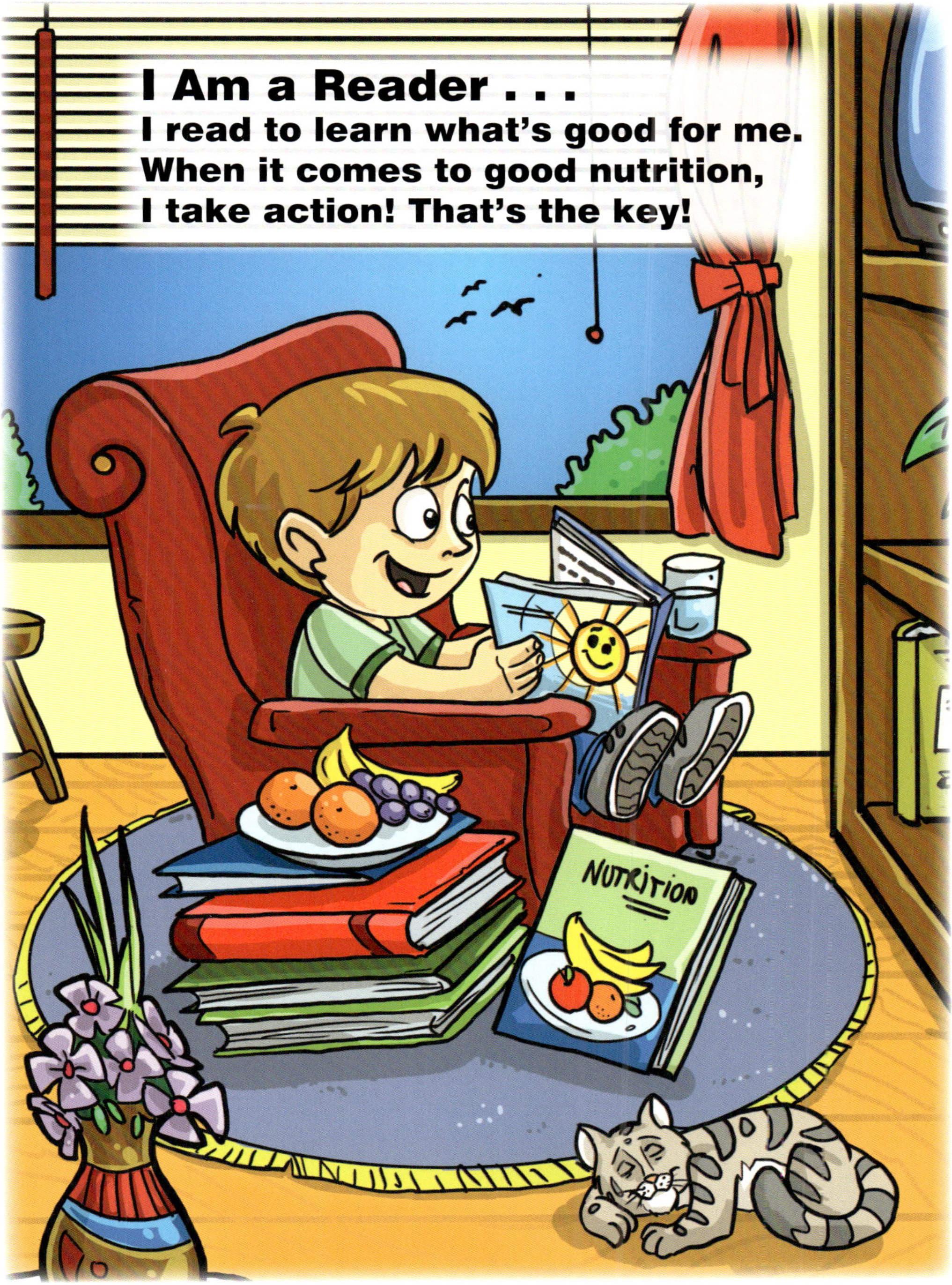

Yo Soy un buen lector...

**Leo para aprender lo que es bueno para mi.
Cuando se trata de una buena nutrición,
tomar acción! Es la clave!**

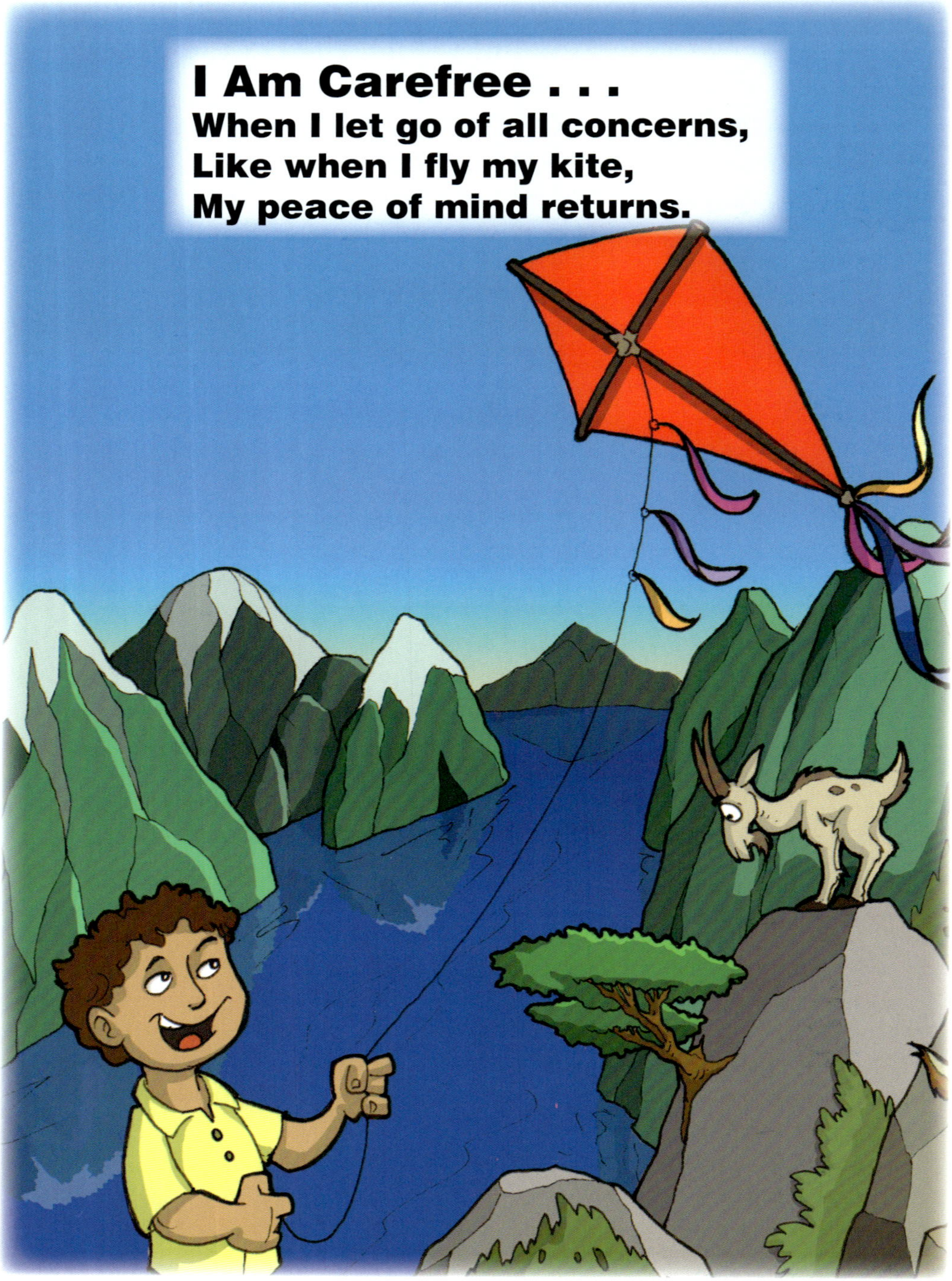
I Am Carefree . . .
When I let go of all concerns,
Like when I fly my kite,
My peace of mind returns.

Yo Soy Despreocupado...

**Cuando dejo atrás todas mis preocupaciones,
como cuando vuelo mi cometa,
mi paz mental regresa.**

I Am Quiet . . .

When I take time for me,
I take time to be still,
And take a deep breath, or two, or three.

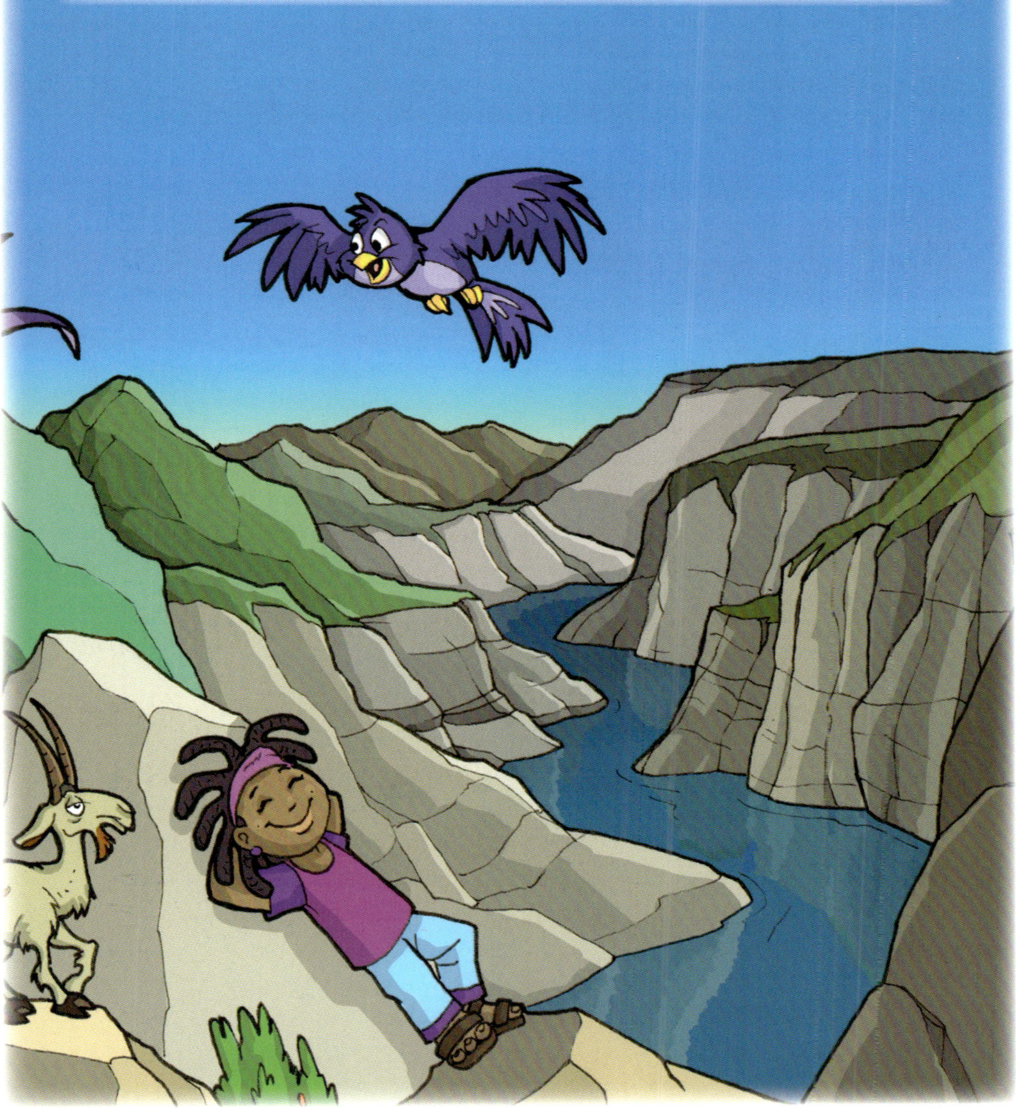

Yo Soy Tranquilo...

Cuando tomo tiempo para mí,
lo tomo para estar tranquilo.
Y respiro hondo una vez, o dos, o tres.

I Am Music!

Feeling the sounds inside my soul.
I love to sing and dance,
Making me happy, joyful, and whole.

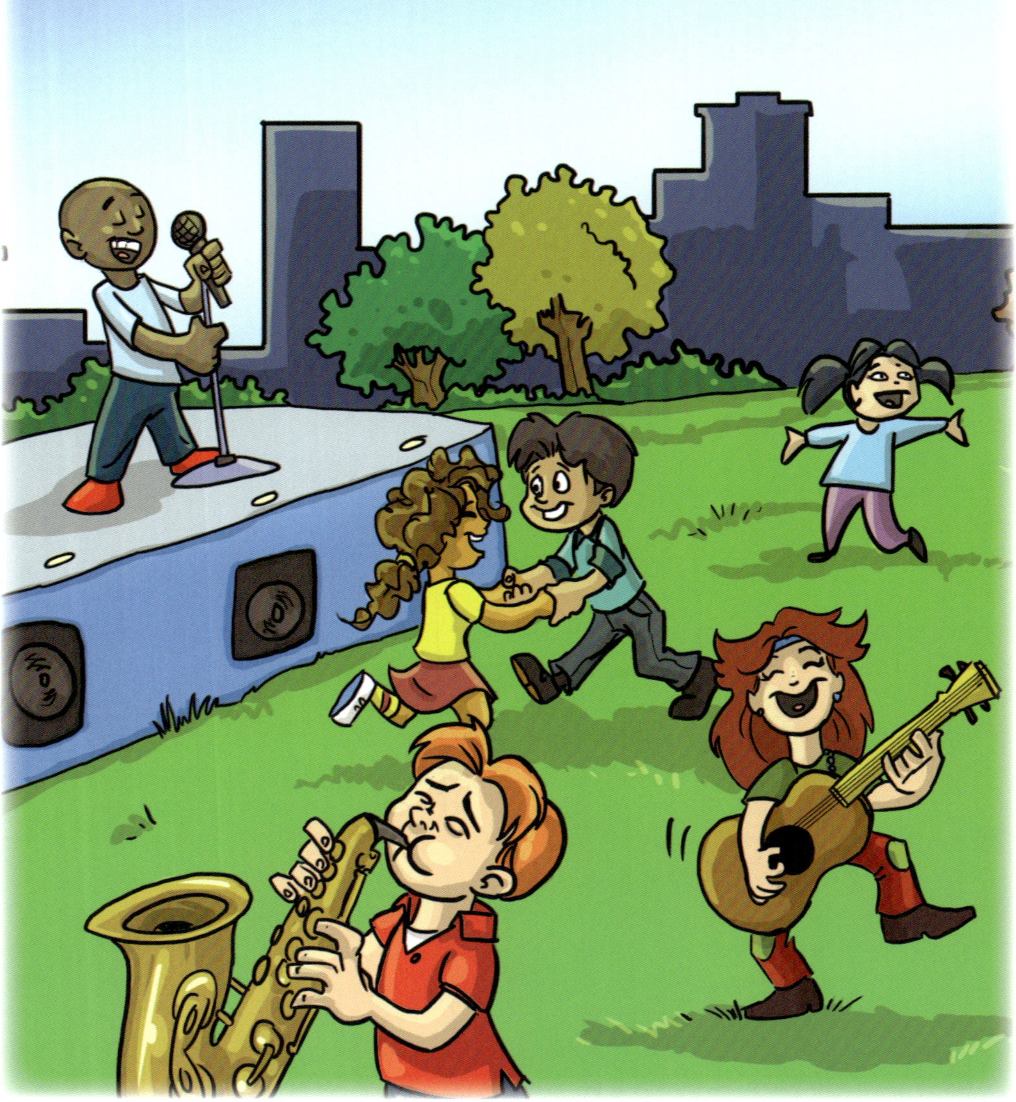

Yo soy Música!

Y siento los sonidos dentro de mi alma.
Me encanta cantar y bailar,
haciéndome feliz, alegre y completo.

I Am Laughter!

And what a joy it is to know,
That every time I laugh,
I feel good from head to toe.

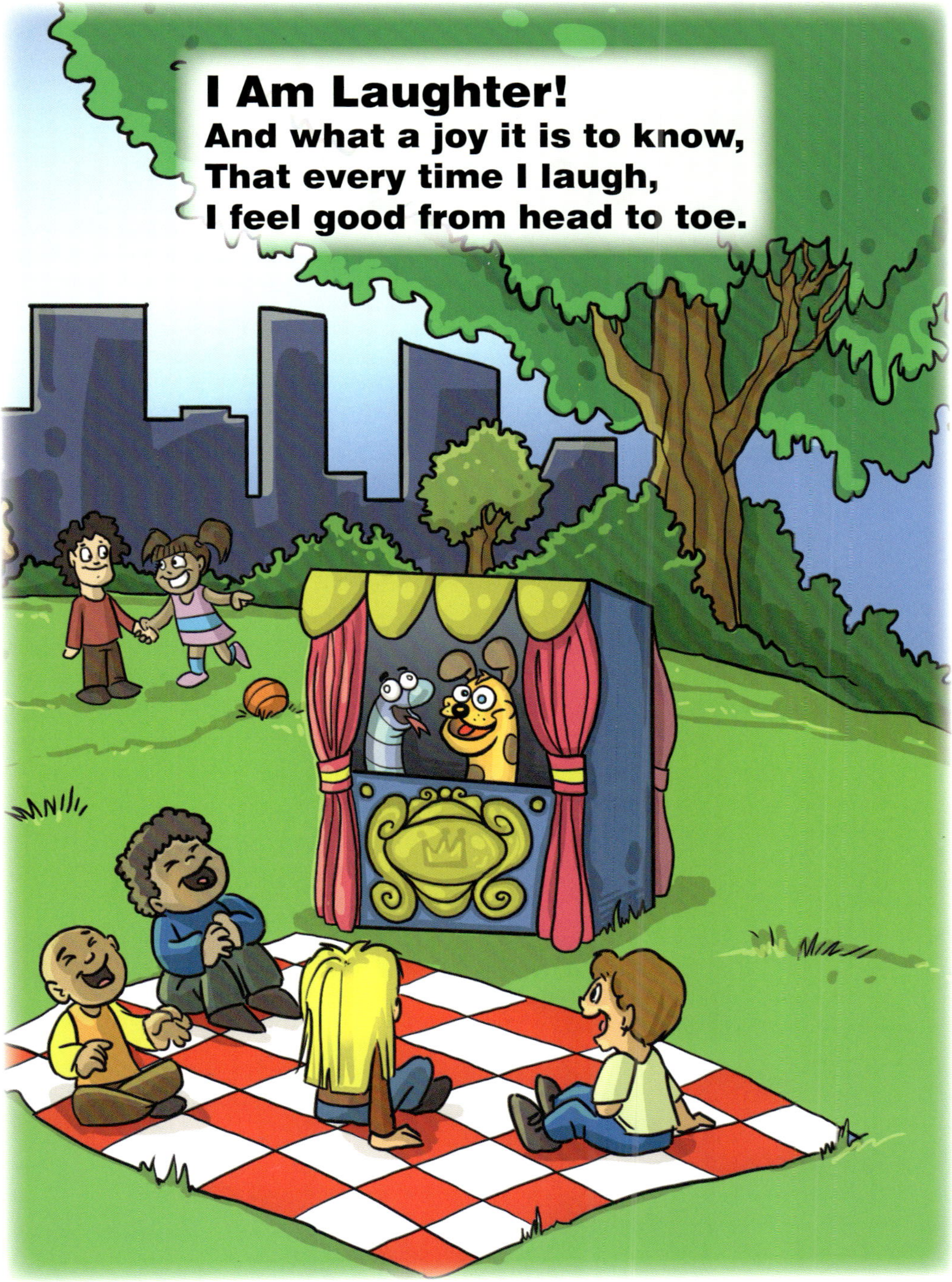

Yo Soy la Risa!

Y qué alegría es saber,
que cada vez que río,
me siento bien de la cabeza a los pies.

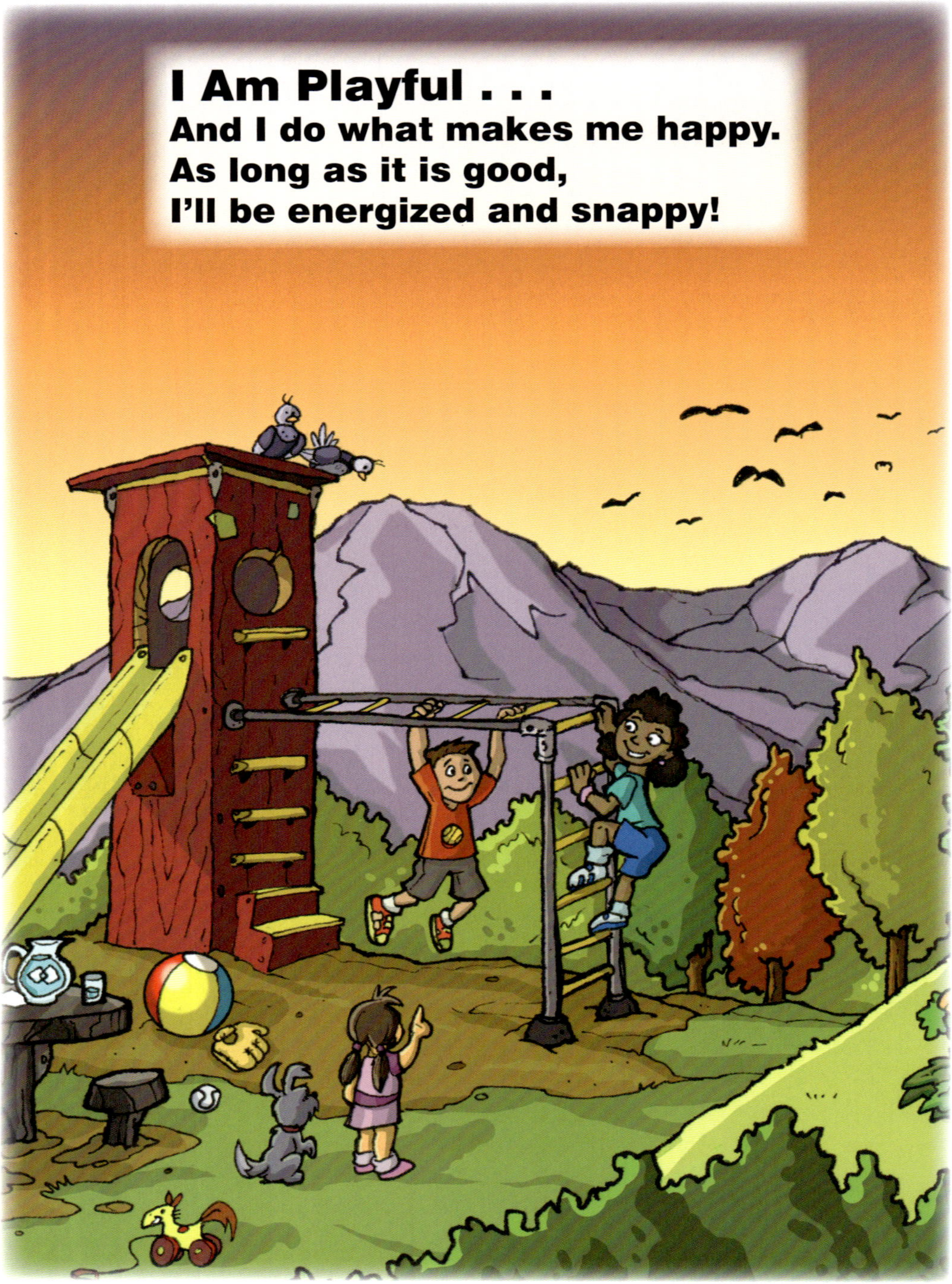
I Am Playful . . .
And I do what makes me happy.
As long as it is good,
I'll be energized and snappy!

Yo Soy Juguetón...

Y hago lo que me hace feliz.
Mientras sea bueno,
me vigoriza y da energía

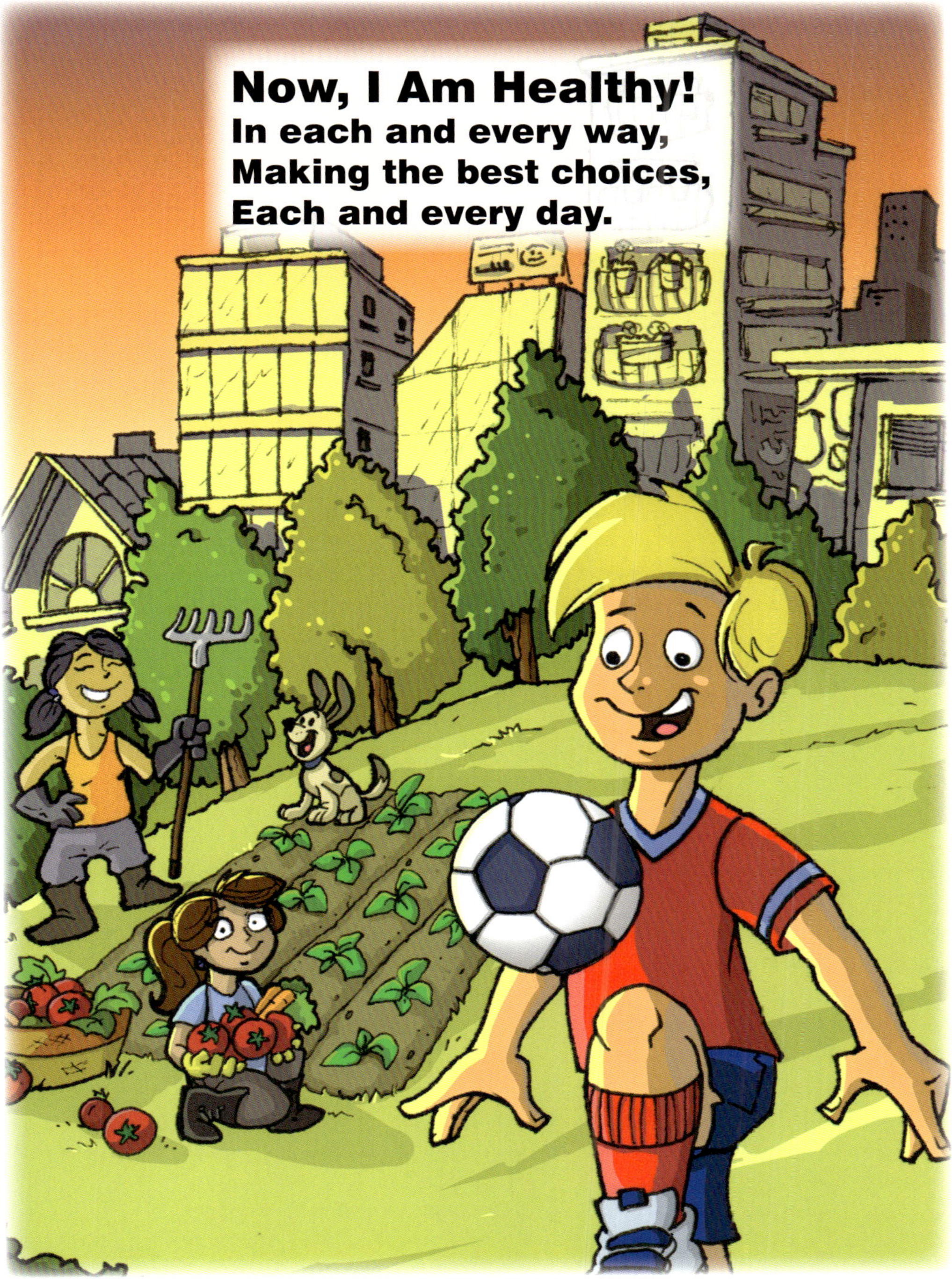
Now, I Am Healthy!
In each and every way,
Making the best choices,
Each and every day.

Ahora, Yo Soy Sano!

En cada uno y todos los sentidos.
Tomando las mejores decisiones,
cada día y todos los días!

Healthy Scoop Workbook Pages

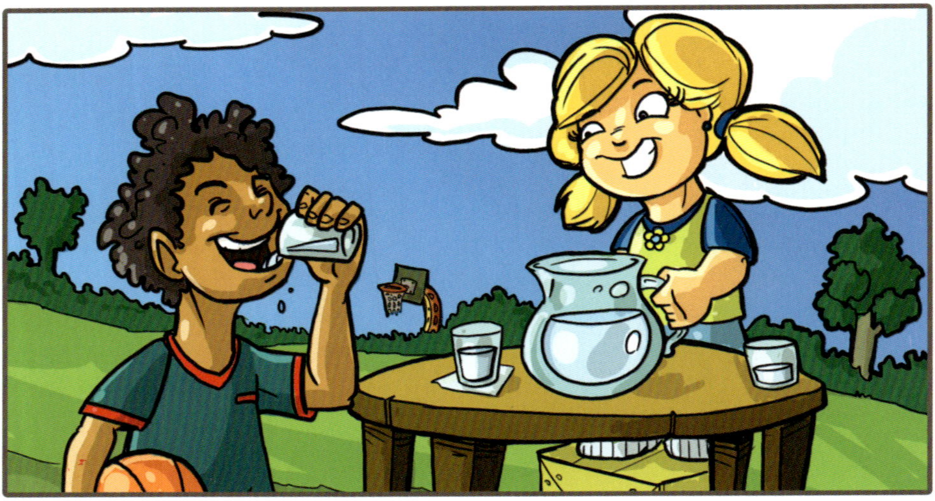

Healthy Scoop

A collection of hands-on, minds-on, hearts-on worksheets developed by **Kid Scoop®** for the ***I Am Healthy!*** book and **The I AM Foundation!**

The book ***I Am Healthy! Affirmations for Health and Well-Being*** provides an extraordinary tool to help teachers easily introduce into the classroom healthy lifestyle choices and character education. When students make healthy choices, the classroom takes on a more-caring atmosphere, and students feel better about themselves. With students better able to absorb and learn, teachers can then effectively reinforce those strategically important concepts for making healthy choices.

Keep the *I Am Healthy!* Affirmations alive in the classroom!

- Each week, have a class ***I Am Healthy!*** Affirmation of the Week chosen from the 22 affirmations in the ***I Am Healthy!*** book.
- Write the ***I Am Healthy!*** Affirmation of the Week on the chalk board.
- With the entire class, recite, aloud, an ***I Am Healthy!*** Affirmation of the Week, one or more times a day.
- Encourage students to memorize the ***I Am Healthy!*** Affirmation of the Week.
- Have students make an ***I Am Healthy***! Affirmation-of-the-Week poster.
- Read, aloud, the affirmations on the beautifully illustrated pages of the ***I Am Healthy!*** book.
- Re-read the ***I Am Healthy!*** Affirmation on each worksheet.
- Complete the worksheet that goes with the ***I Am Healthy!*** Affirmation of the Week.
- Share the worksheet activity with a friend or family member.
- Encourage students to catch a classmate in an action that reflects the ***I Am Healthy!*** Affirmation of the week.

An award-winning educational publisher, Kid Scoop® publications include the weekly Kid Scoop® syndicated newspaper feature for kids, which appears in more than 300 newspapers and websites. **www.kidscoop.com**

Paginas del Libro de Trabajo: Scoop de la Salud

Scoop de la Salud

Una colección de manos a la obra, y corazones a las hojas de trabajo creadas por **Kid Scoop®** para el libro **¡Yo Soy Sano!** y **¡La Fundación Yo Soy!**

• El libro ***¡Yo Soy Sano! Afirmaciones de Salud y Bienestar*** proporciona una herramienta extraordinaria para ayudar a los Maestros a introducir fácilmente en el salón de clase las opciones de un estilo de vida sano y educación de carácter. Cuando los estudiantes toman decisiones saludables, el ambiente del salón de clases se convierte en un lugar con una atmósfera mas agradable y los maestros pueden reforzar eficazmente esos conceptos estratégicamente importantes para elegir opciones sanas.

¡A mantener las Afirmaciones ¡Yo Soy Sano! vivas en el salón de clases!

- Cada semana, tengan una clase de ***¡Yo-Soy Sano!*** Afirmaciones de la Semana escogidas de las 22 afirmaciones de el libro ***¡Yo Soy Sano!***
- Escriban la Afirmación de ***¡Yo Soy Sano!*** de la semana en el pizarrón
- Que toda la clase repita, en voz alta, la Afirmación que hayan escogido en la semana ***¡Yo Soy Sano!*** una o mas veces al día.
- Alentar a los estudiantes a memorizar su Afirmación ***¡Yo Soy Sano!*** de la semana.
- Haga que los estudiantes creen un poster de- la- Afirmación de la Semana ***¡Yo Soy Sano!***
- Lea en voz alta, las Afirmaciones de las paginas bellamente ilustradas de el libro ***¡Yo Soy Sano!***
- Releer la Afirmación ***¡Yo Soy Sano!*** en cada hoja de trabajo
- Complete la hoja de trabajo que corresponde a la Afirmación ***¡Yo Soy Sano!*** de la Semana.
- Compartir la hoja de trabajo con un miembro de su familia o amigo.
- Anime a sus estudiantes a tomar por sorpresa a un compañero de clase en una acción que refleje la Afirmación ***¡Yo Soy Sano!*** de la semana.

Publicaciones Kid Scoop® es una editorial educativa galardonada. Niño Scoop ®incluye el periódico sindicado semanal Kid Scoop® de niños, que aparece en más de 300 periódicos y sitios web. **www.kidscoop.com**

I Am Fitness!
And when I excercise each day,
I love the way I feel.
Feeling joy along the way.

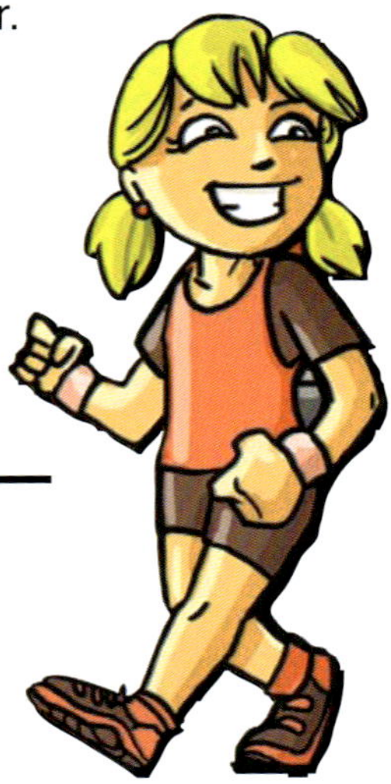

Use a **penny** or a **small button** as a marker. Flip your marker onto the hopscotch chart. You must land on the first box and do that activity before you can go on to the second box, and so on.

Can you do all 7 fitness activities?

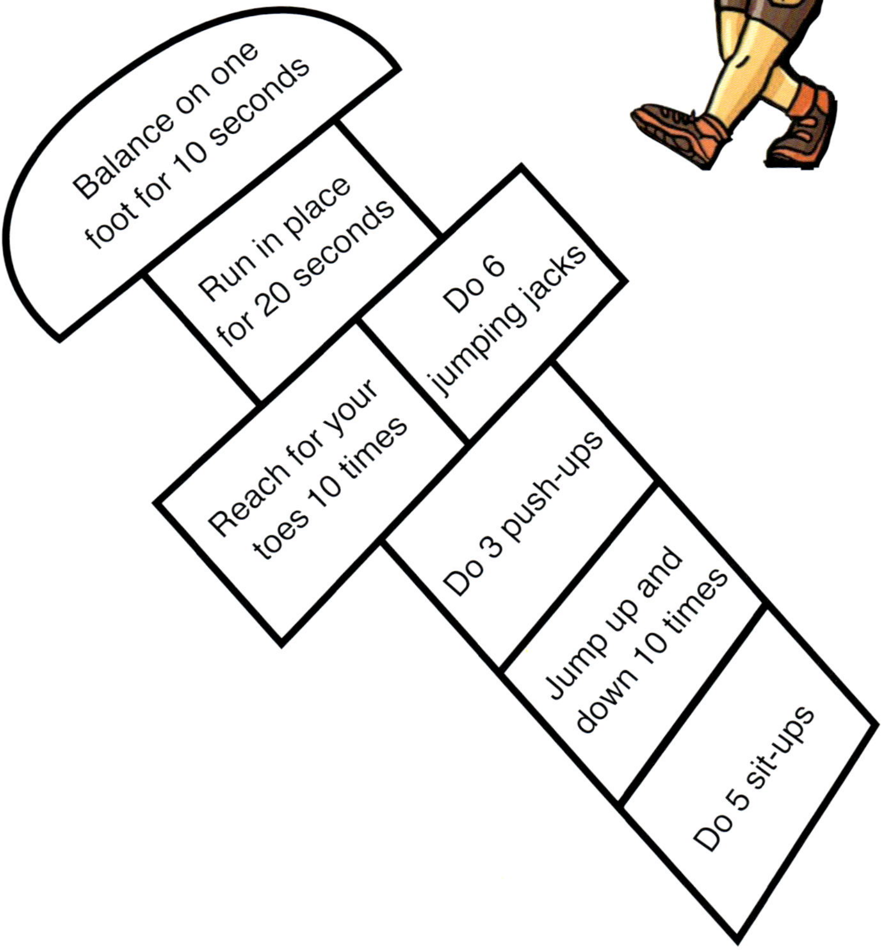
Balance on one foot for 10 seconds
Run in place for 20 seconds
Do 6 jumping jacks
Reach for your toes 10 times
Do 3 push-ups
Jump up and down 10 times
Do 5 sit-ups

Yo Soy y estoy en buen estado físico!
Y cuando me ejercito cada día,
Me encanta como me siento.
Y esa alegría guía mi camino.

Utiliza un **centavo** ó un **botón pequeño** como marcador. Tira tu marcador en la ilustración de la rayuela. Tiene que aterrizar en el primer cuadro y hacer esa actividad antes de ir al segundo cuadro y así sucesivamente.

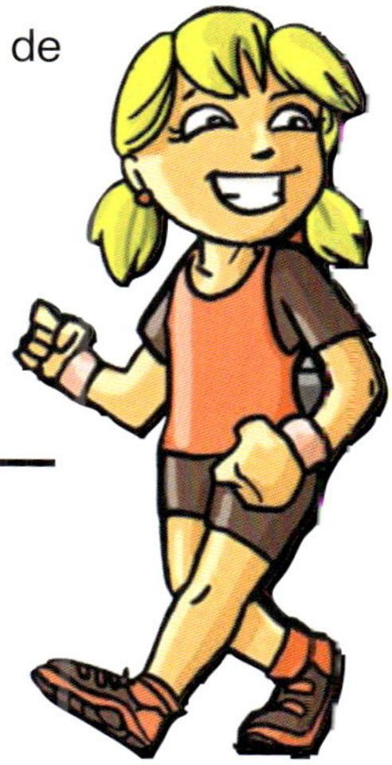

Puedes ejercitar estas 7 actividades?

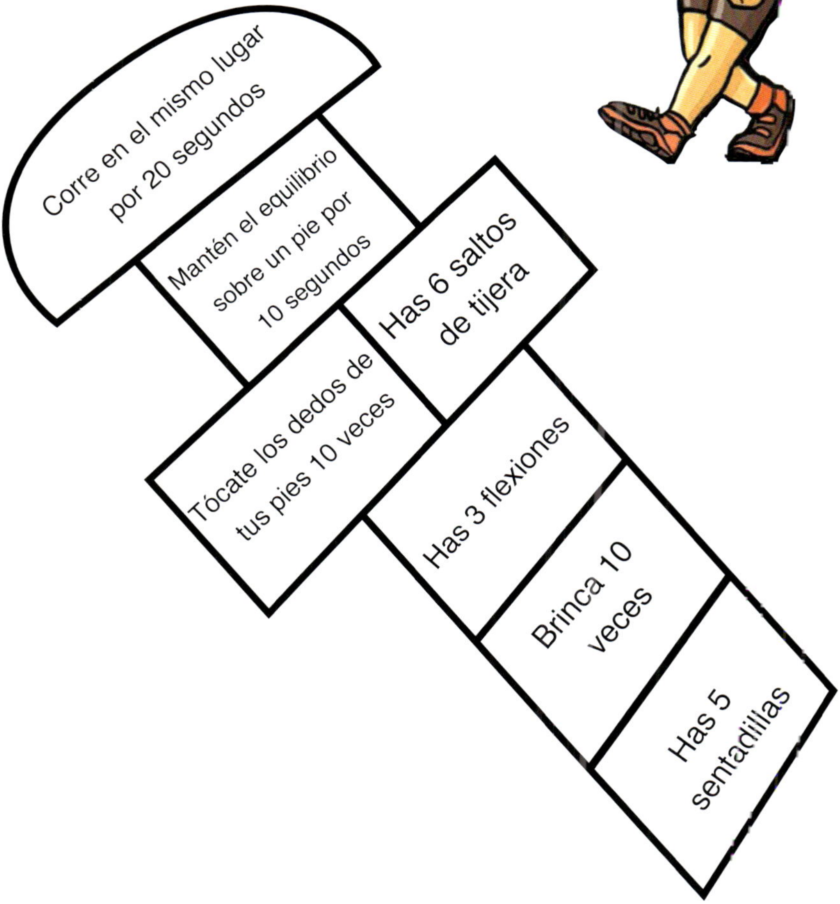

I Am Friendly!
Making friends while having fun,
One of the keys to my success,
So I can easily get things done.

10 Steps to Friendship

For each letter on the ladder, write something nice that friends do for each other.

F

R

I

E

N

D

S

H

I

P

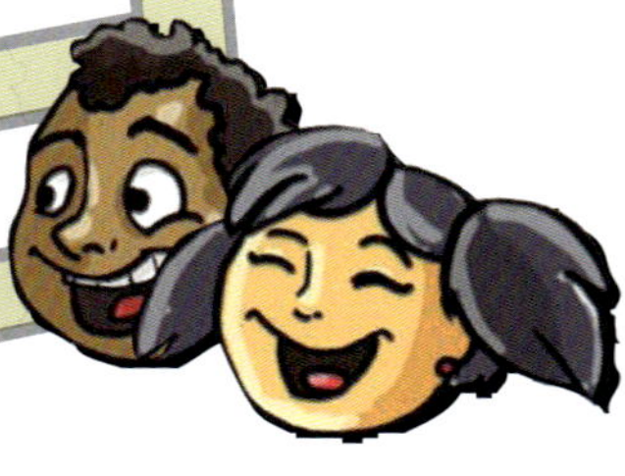

Yo Soy amigable...
Haciendo amigos mientras me divierto,
una de las claves de mi éxito,
Para terminar de hacer las cosas fácilmente.

10 pasos hacia la Amistad

Por cada una de las letras, escribe algo de lo bueno que hacen los amigos unos a otros.

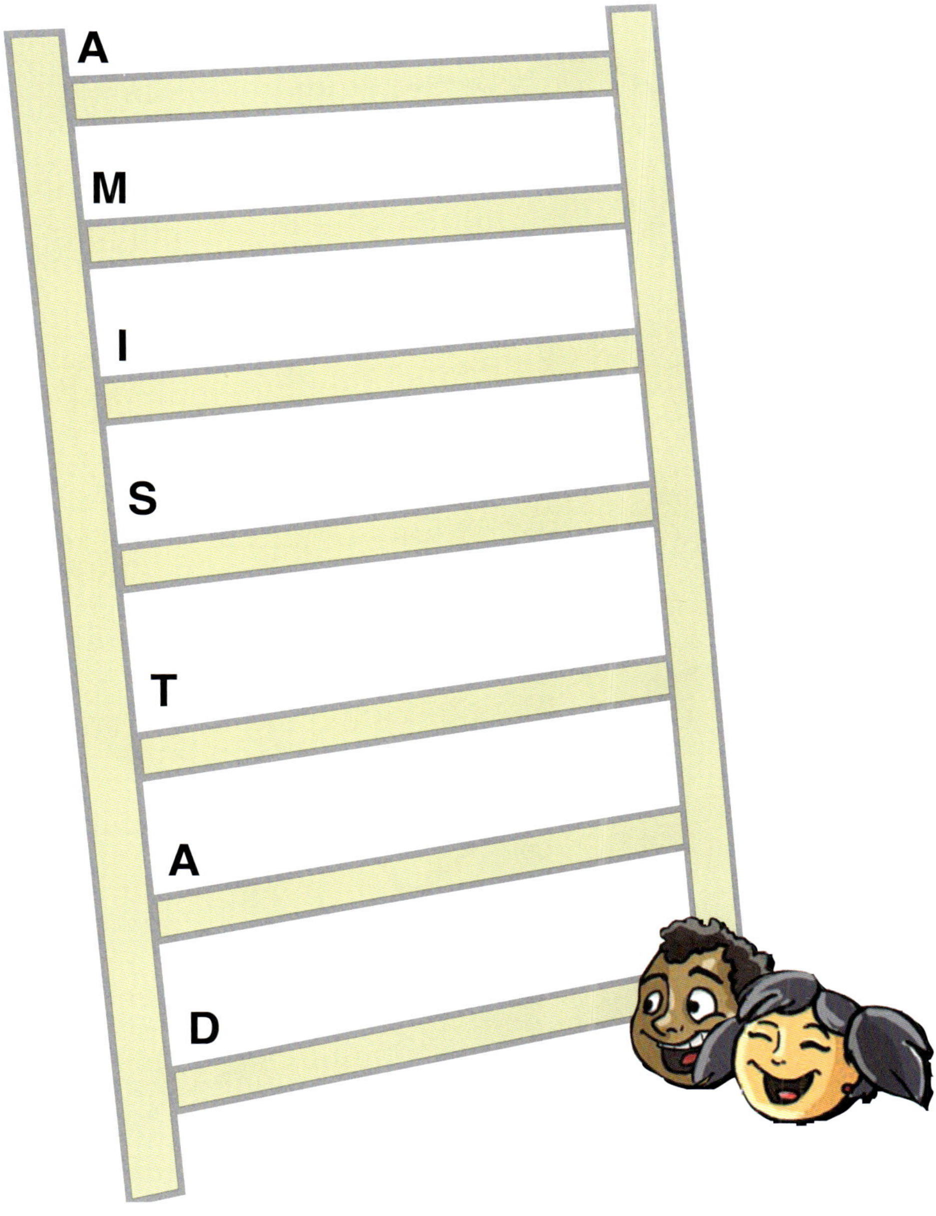

I Am Active!
I love to exercise my heart.
When I run, swim, or walk,
My health soars off the chart!

Each time you do an activity in one of the hearts, color the heart!

Play catch

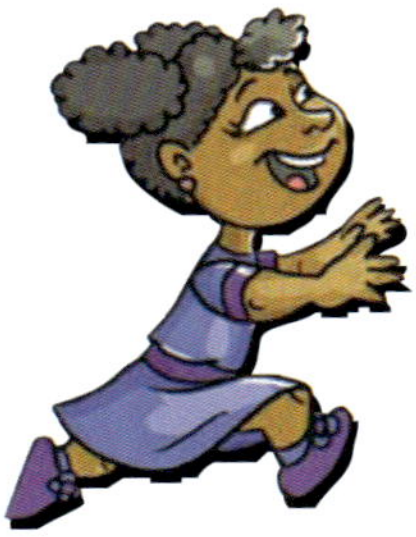

Do 5 jumping jacks

Jump rope

Run for a minute

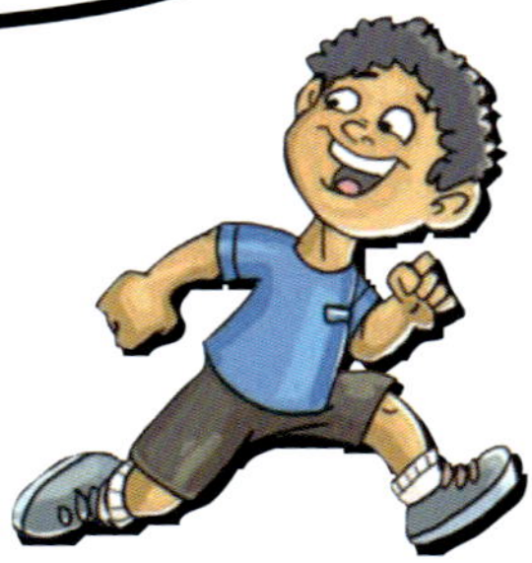

Hop like a bunny

Dance in your room

Crawl like a snake

Yo soy Activo!
Me encanta ejercitar mi corazón.
Cuando corro, nado, o paseo
mi salud es fuera de serie!

Jugar a atrapar

Cada que termines cada actividad, colorea el corazón

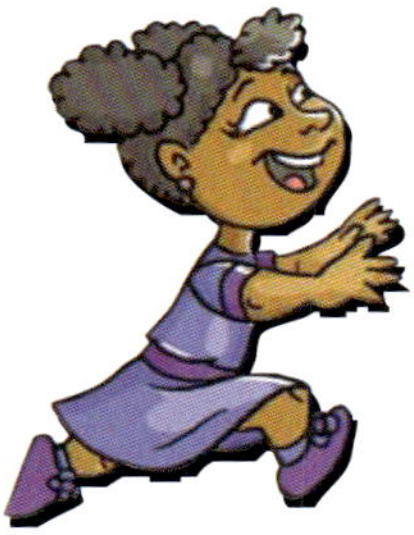

Brinca 3 veces

Corre por un minuto

Brinca la cuerda

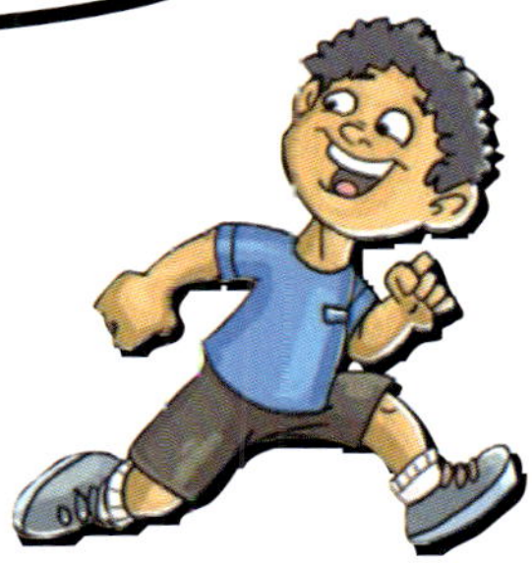

Brinca de conejito

Baila en tu cuarto

Arrástrate como serpiente

I Am Happy!
Surrounded by good friends,
Relaxing and having fun, and
Being together on weekends.

What makes you happy?
Draw a picture of yourself
when you're happy.

Portrait of ____________________

Yo Soy Feliz!
Y rodeado de buenos amigos.
Me relajo y me divierto,
junto con ellos los fines de semana.

Que te hace feliz?
Haz un dibujo de ti
cuando estas feliz.

Retrato de ____________________

I Am Energy!
Daily I give gratitude
For all the good things in my life
Giving me my positive attitude.

Grateful Morning, Noon and Night

On the lines below, write something you are grateful for in the morning, at noon, and at night.

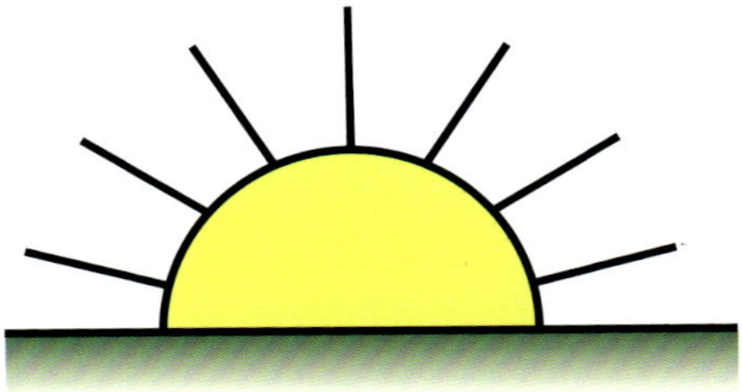

Morning: ______________________

____

____

____

____

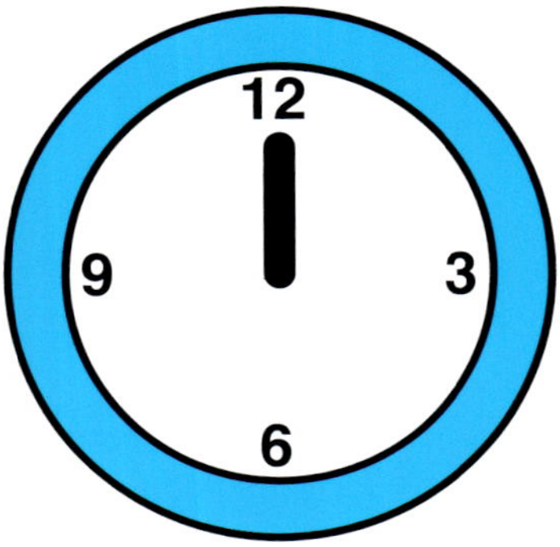

Noon: ______________________

____

____

____

____

Night: ______________________

____

____

____

____

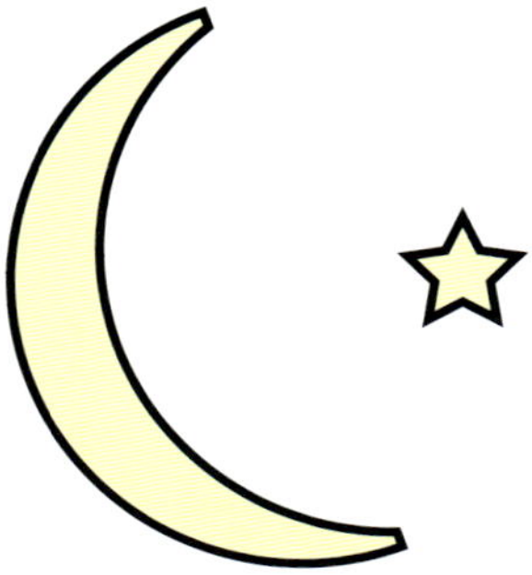

Yo Soy Energia!
Diariamente doy gracias
Por todas las cosas buenas en mi vida
Y me doy a mi mismo una actitud positivo.

Agradecido mañana, tarde y noche

En las líneas de abajo, escribe algo de lo que estés agradecido por la mañana, tarde y noche.

Mañana: ______________________________

____

____

____

____

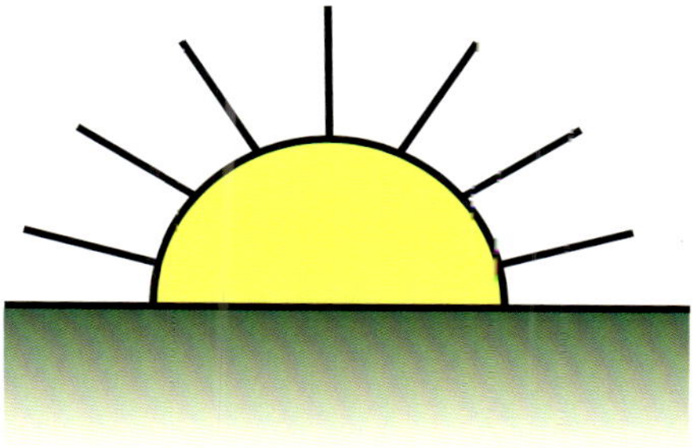

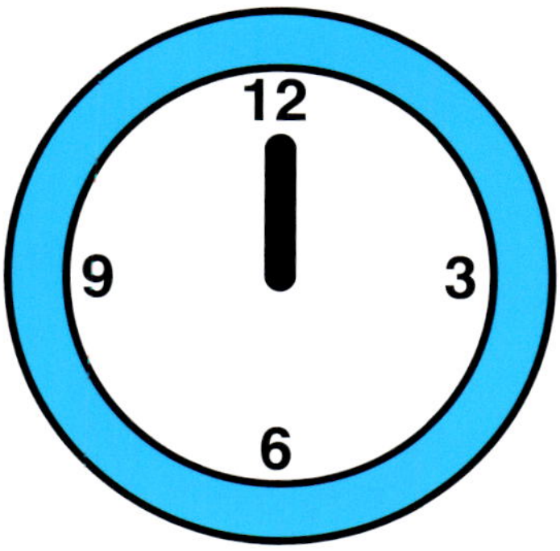

Tarde: ______________________________

____

____

____

____

Noche: ______________________________

____

____

____

____

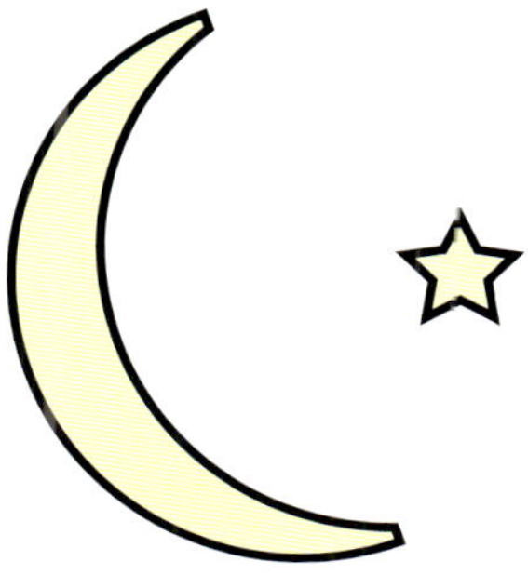

I Am Joyful!
So I jump for joy,
When I play outside...
Like enjoying my favorite toy.

Find Your Pulse and Jump for Joy!

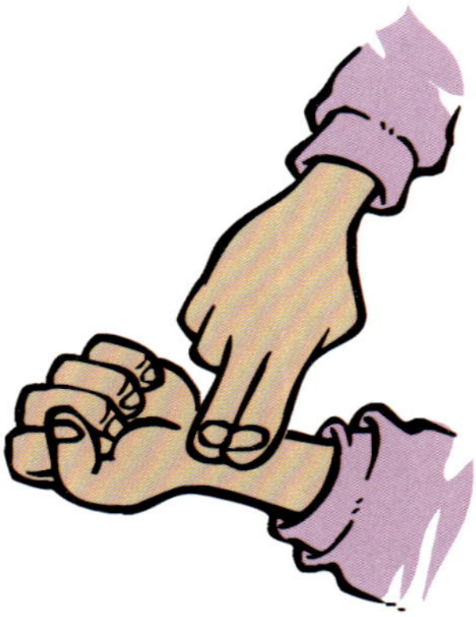

Find your **pulse** by lightly pressing on the skin anywhere there's a large artery running just beneath your skin. Two good places to find it are on the side of your neck and the inside of your wrist, just below the thumb.

You'll know that you've found your pulse when you can feel a small beat under your skin.

Use a watch with a second hand, and count how many beats you feel in one minute. This is your **resting heartbeat.**

My resting heart beat is ________ beats per minute.

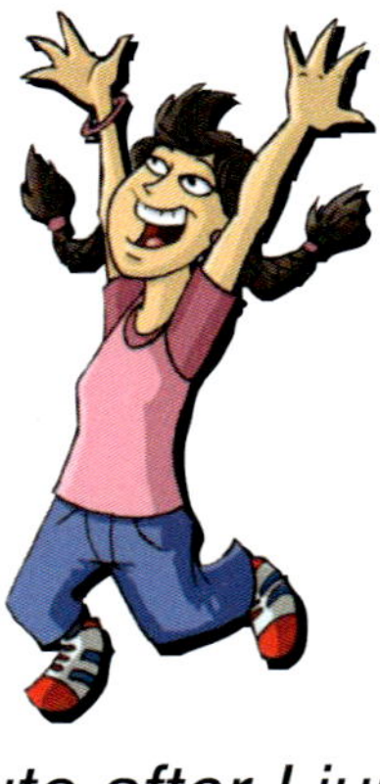

Try hopping up and down for one minute and taking your pulse again – now how many beats do you count in one minute?

My heart beats _____ times per minute after I jump around for a minute.

Yo Soy Alegre!
Por lo tanto brinco de alegría,
Cuando salgo a jugar afuera,
Es como si disfrutara mi juguete favorito.

Encuentra tu pulso y brinca de alegría

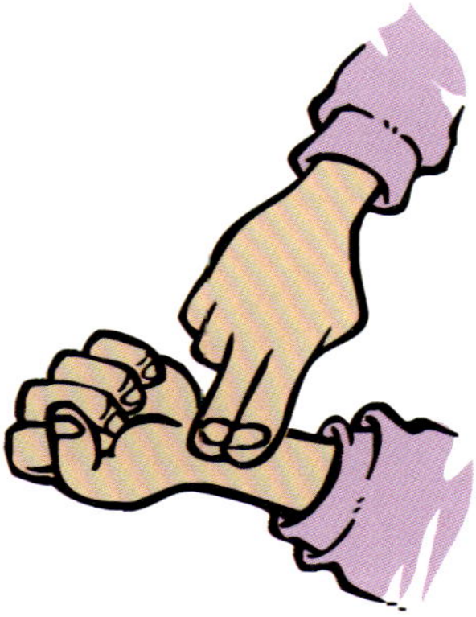

Encuentra tu pulso presionando suavemente la piel endonde encuentres la vena larga que corre bajo tu piel. Dos de los lugares en donde lo encuentras es en el cuello y en tu muñeca exactamente abajo de tu dedo pulgar.

Sabrás que has encontrado tu pulso cuando sientas un pequeño latido bajo tu piel.

Usa el segundero del reloj para contar
cuantos latidos sientes en un minuto.
Este es el **latido de tu corazón**

El pulso de mi corazón es ________ latidos por minuto.

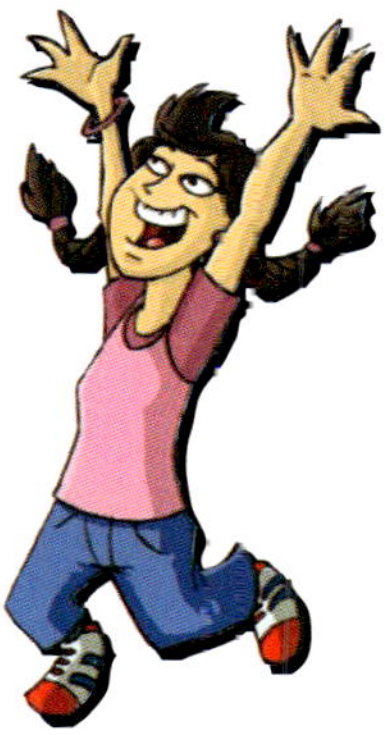

Brinca de arriba abajo por un minute
Y toma tu pulso otra vez- ahora
cuantos latidos contaste en un minuto?

Mi corazón late _____ veces por minuto después de brincar.

I Am Wholeness!
Feeling great about myself
And the body I've been given,
I'm a picture of great health.

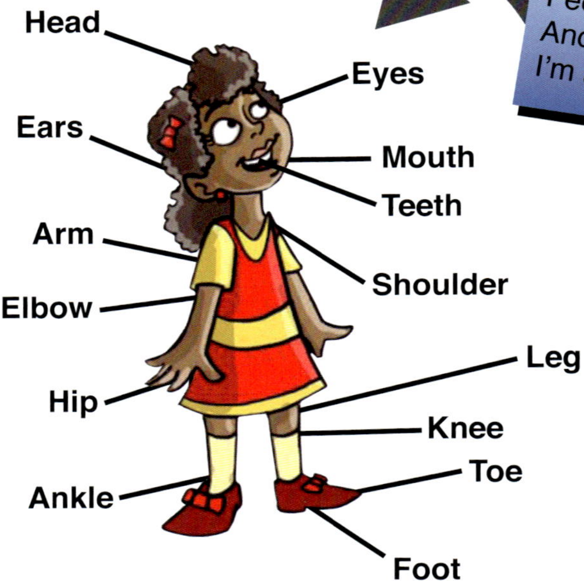

Find each body part in the Word Search.

M	Q	Y	M	O	U	T	H	X	N	E	C	L	E	G
U	B	P	F	O	O	T	V	Q	P	V	S	V	Q	C
T	Z	O	S	Z	X	K	C	V	V	Q	Z	H	C	F
W	E	C	G	V	N	G	D	C	E	K	E	I	I	Z
S	Y	F	R	U	T	A	R	M	A	J	E	P	N	G
H	K	G	O	V	O	W	B	K	R	R	A	V	N	L
Z	P	Z	A	R	U	T	R	H	I	H	R	U	V	T
A	N	K	L	E	Y	E	W	S	Q	S	S	I	M	B
F	K	N	U	K	O	E	S	H	Q	D	N	W	E	A
E	C	E	H	Y	T	T	T	O	E	B	Q	U	L	J
E	Y	E	S	L	C	H	T	U	B	R	L	V	B	H
U	D	E	L	Q	E	G	L	L	S	W	F	D	O	E
X	F	E	V	Q	S	E	U	D	E	X	X	Z	W	A
P	U	T	J	H	A	O	O	E	T	M	Q	S	J	D
B	U	B	T	H	C	M	Y	R	G	J	Y	V	V	C

Yo Soy Plenitud!
Sintiéndome bien conmigo mismo
Y con el cuerpo que se me ha dado,
Soy la viva imagen de la salud

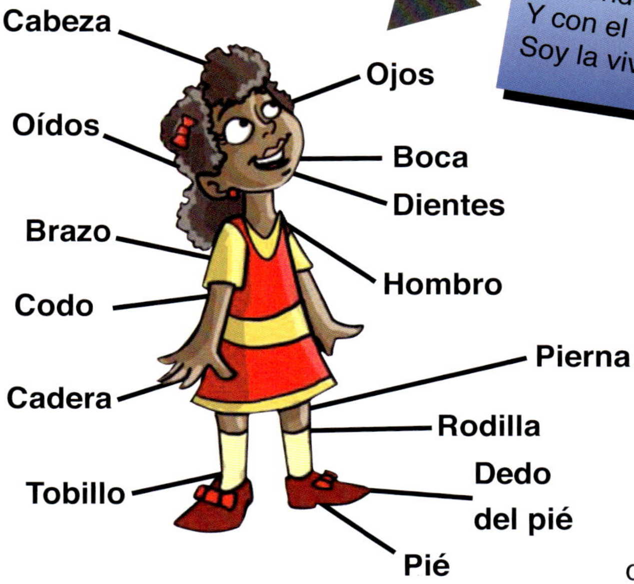

Encuentra las palabras por cada parte del cuerpo.

K	H	I	O	Y	X	B	J	L	M	E	Q	U	Z	F
Z	V	O	G	R	V	R	N	A	C	O	U	X	O	O
C	W	O	L	X	B	M	N	S	M	N	R	C	S	R
A	B	Y	A	A	G	M	E	V	L	T	G	O	N	O
D	G	T	R	N	P	T	O	A	Z	J	S	D	P	F
E	Q	N	S	R	N	O	B	H	W	S	Z	O	F	L
R	P	E	Y	E	V	N	L	N	Z	L	D	R	F	I
A	U	J	I	I	O	A	P	L	W	L	B	Z	S	E
V	H	D	Q	P	A	Z	B	P	I	W	S	O	D	O
D	M	M	Q	L	I	T	A	U	M	B	J	D	Y	Z
V	F	H	V	L	H	O	Z	R	F	O	O	X	I	B
L	J	P	F	O	J	R	B	M	B	A	G	T	K	M
W	T	K	G	H	X	O	P	S	P	S	Z	X	E	E
Q	L	H	J	D	C	I	J	X	V	T	V	F	F	X
K	A	W	V	A	Z	H	A	Z	E	B	A	C	E	U

I Am Consistent!
Going to the dentist or the doc,
Getting regular check-ups,
So my health runs like a clock.

Brush your teeth every day at least two or three times.

Be consistent!

1. Find a brushing buddy at home.

2. Ask your buddy to color a star in the correct box each time you brush your teeth. Can you earn at least two stars daily?

Sunday	Monday	Tuesday	Wednesday	Thursday	Friday	Saturday

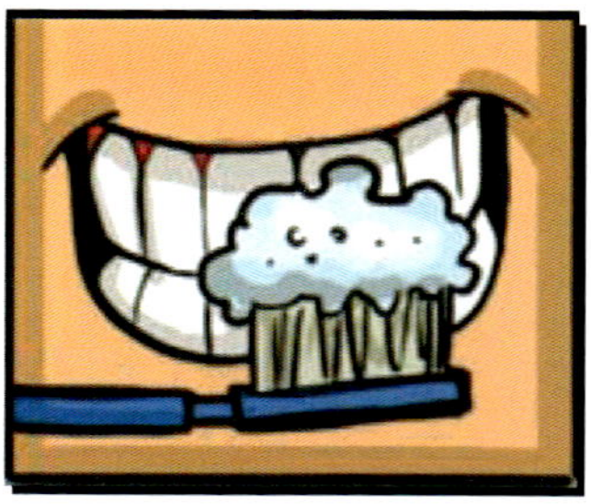

Yo Soy Consistente!
Cuando visito al dentista o al doctor,
y me checo regularmente,
mi salud funciona como un reloj.

Cepilla tus dientes todos los días por lo menos dos o tres veces.

Se consistente!

1. Busca quien se cepille los dientes contigo en casa.

2. Pide a esa persona que colore una estrellita de las que están adentro de la caja cada que te cepilles los dientes. Crees que puedas ganarte por lo menos dos estrellitas diarias?

Domingo	Lunes	Martes	Miércoles	Jueves	Viernes	Sábado

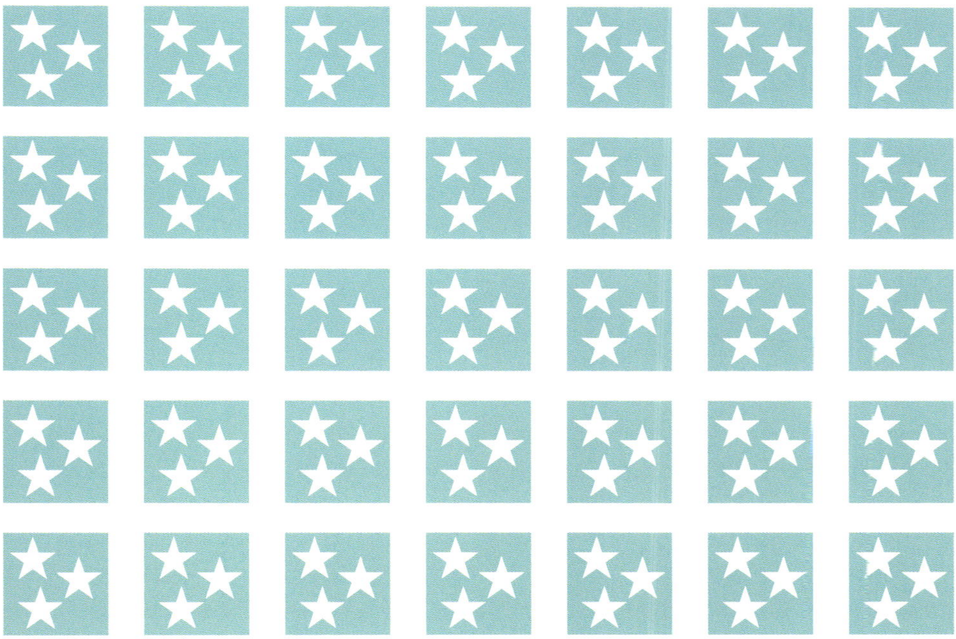

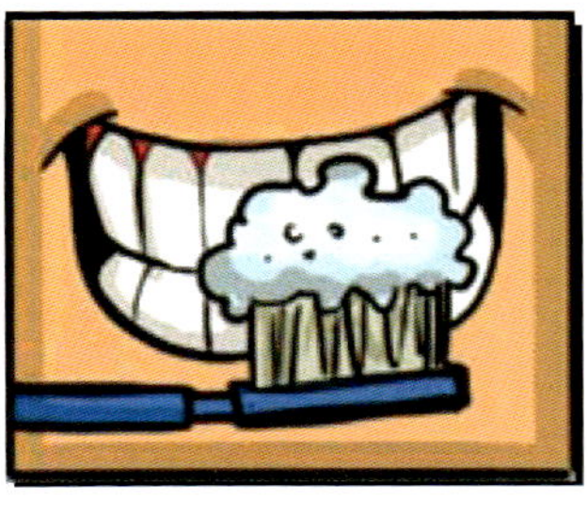

I Am Wise!
I make good choices every day,
Which support my health and well-being.
Now, I'm on my way.

Healthy Choices are Wise Choices

Follow the maze to good health. Along the way there are good choices and choices that are not so good. Make the good choices to get to the Healthy, Happy, Glowing Finish!

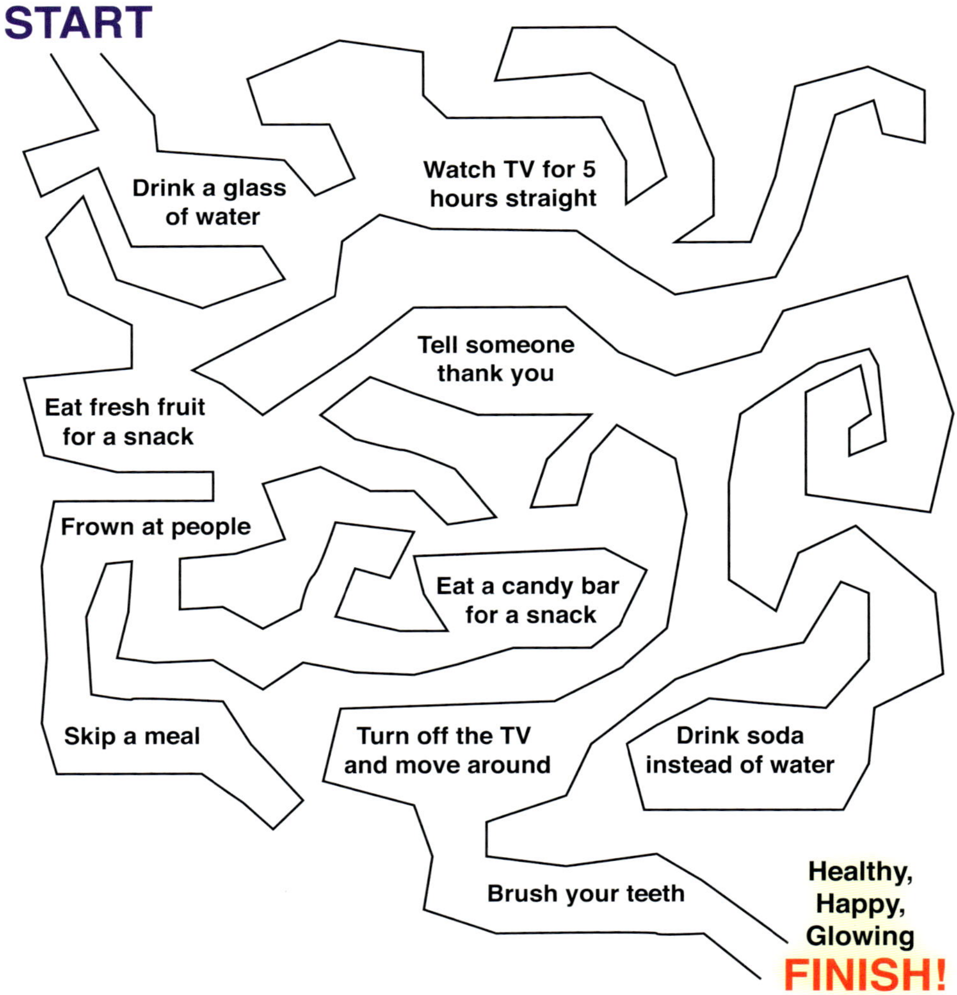

Yo soy sabio!
Y tomo buenas decisiones cada día, y todos los días
Que apoyan mi salud y bienestar
Ahora se el camino a seguir.

Sigue el laberinto de la buena salud. En el encontraras decisiones buenas y otras no tan buenas.Escoge las decisiones que te llevarán al camino de la Salud, Felicidad, y un Final Brillante.

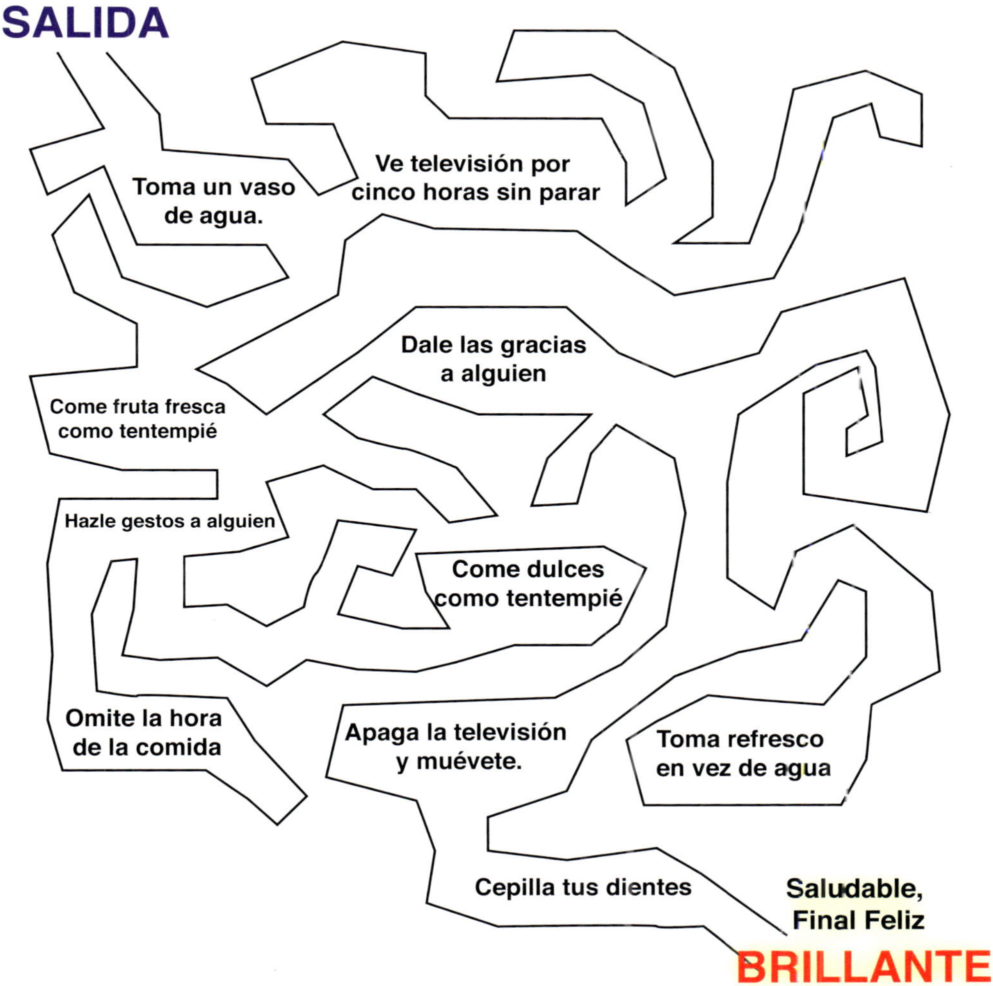

SALIDA
Toma un vaso de agua.
Ve televisión por cinco horas sin parar
Dale las gracias a alguien
Come fruta fresca como tentempié
Hazle gestos a alguien
Come dulces como tentempié
Omite la hora de la comida
Apaga la televisión y muévete.
Toma refresco en vez de agua
Cepilla tus dientes
Saludable, Final Feliz
BRILLANTE

I Am Refreshed!
By the water that I drink,
Which purifies my body.
To my health, water is the link.

Water Wisdom

Do the math under each question, then match it to the answer with the correct math solution.

What part of your body is made up of water?
8 - 3 = ___

How much water do you lose each day?
5 + 1 = ___

How do you replace water in your body?
4 - 2 = ___

What things does water do in our bodies?
9 + 4 = ___

Should you only drink water when you are thirsty?
7 - 4 = ___

(3) ***No. Try to take a drink each time you pass a water fountain.***

(13) ***Keeps your body temperature normal, lubricates and cushions your joints, and protects your spinal cord and other sensitive tissues.***

(6) ***2-3 quarts***

(5) ***60%***

(2) ***By eating juicy foods and drinking water.***

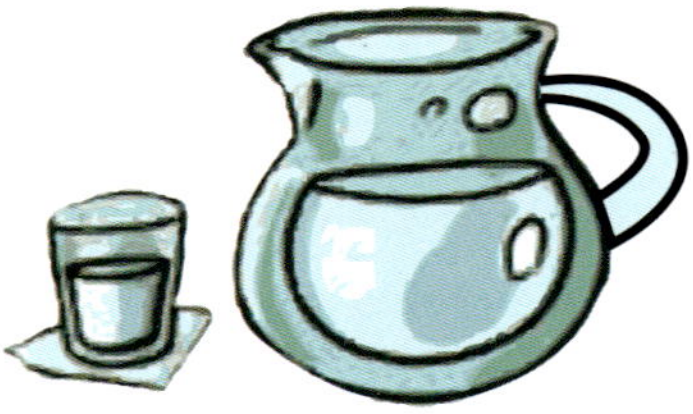

Fill a glass with water. Count how many swallows it takes to drink the whole cup! Try this with different-sized cups.

Yo Soy y me siento fresco!
Por que el agua que tomo,
Purifica mi cuerpo
El agua es el enlace para mi salud

Agua Sabiduría

Haz las cuentas para que descubras las respuestas a cada pregunta.

Que parte de tu cuerpo esta hecho de agua?
8 - 3 = ____

Cuanta agua pierdes por cada día?
5 + 1 = ____

Como reemplazas agua en tu cuerpo?
4 - 2 = ____

Que es lo que hace el agua en nuestros cuerpos?
9 + 4 = ____

Debes de tomar agua solo cuando tienes sed?
7 - 4 = ____

(3) ***No. Trata de tomar un trago cada vez que pasas por una fuente.***

(13) ***Mantiene la temperatura normal,lubrica y amortigua articulaciones, y protege la médula espinal y otros tejidos sensibles.***

(6) ***2-3 cuartos de galón***

(5) ***60%***

(2) ***lo logras con comidas jugosas y tomando agua.***

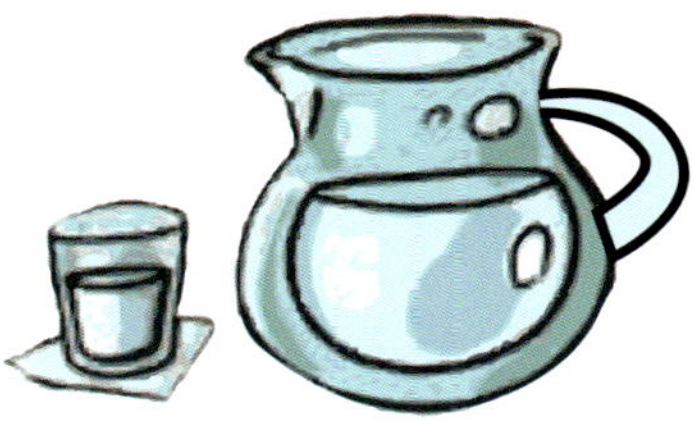

Llena un vaso de agua y cuenta cuantos tragos te tomas para completar el vaso. Prueba hacerlo con diferentes tamaños de vasos.

Nature Walk Notebook

I Am Nature!
I love to hike and walk
To see the sights and hear the sounds
Maybe from a wise, old owl or hawk.

Take a walk outside and use your senses. Then complete the nature notebook page below.

What I saw

What I smelled

What I heard

What I tasted

What I touched and how it felt

Cuaderno de mis caminatas En la naturaleza

Yo soy Naturaleza...
Me ecanta ir de excursión y caminar
Ver los lugares de interés y escuchar los sonidos
Tal vez de un búho viejo y sabio, o de un halcón

Ve de paseo y usa tus sentidos.

Después completa la pagina de tu cuaderno de notas.

Que vi

Que olí

Que oí

Que probé

Que toqué y cómo se siente

I Am Pure!
And like a flowing stream
Inside an incredible forest,
My health is like a dream.

Keep the flowing stream pure and clean.
Cross out the 6 things that don't belong.

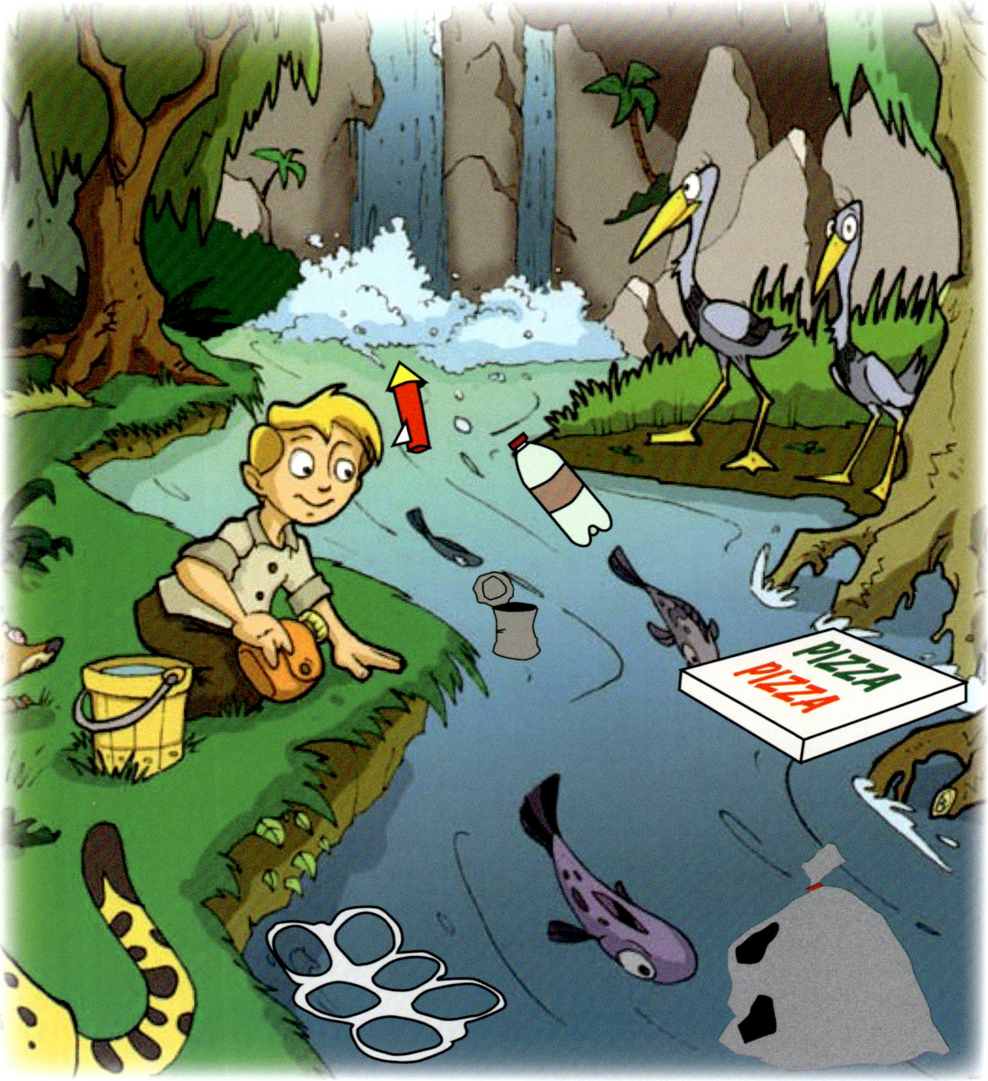

(pizza box, rocket toy, can, bottle,
garbage bag, plastic can-holder)

Yo soy Puro...
Como la corriente que fluye
Dentro de un bosque increíble,
Mi salud es como un sueño.

Mantén el riachuelo puro y limpio.
Tacha las 6 cosas que no pertenecen al riachuelo

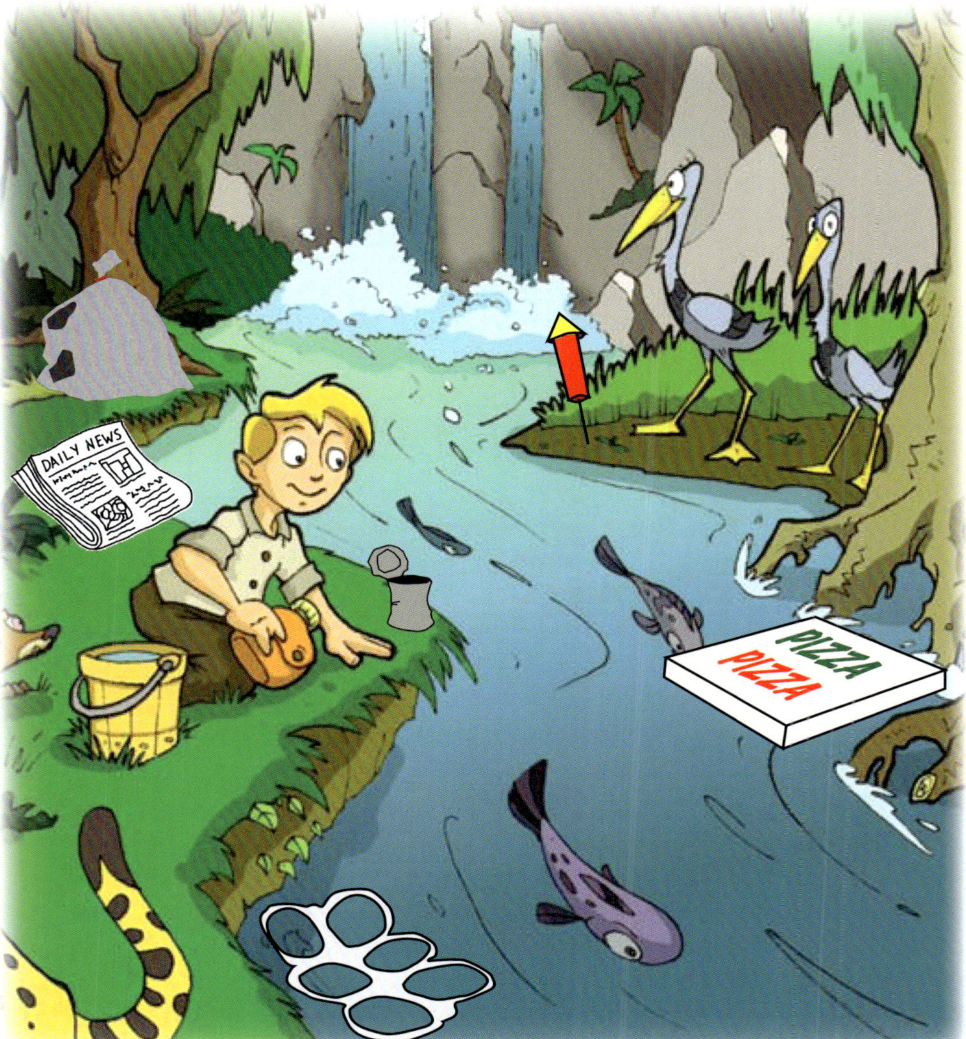

Caja de pizza, juguete, lata, botella, bolsa de basura, sostenedor de refresco en lata.

I Am All Natural!
And I create a healthy me.
Choosing nature's snacks and treats,
Like an apple from a tree!

Draw a healthy snack
on your plate.

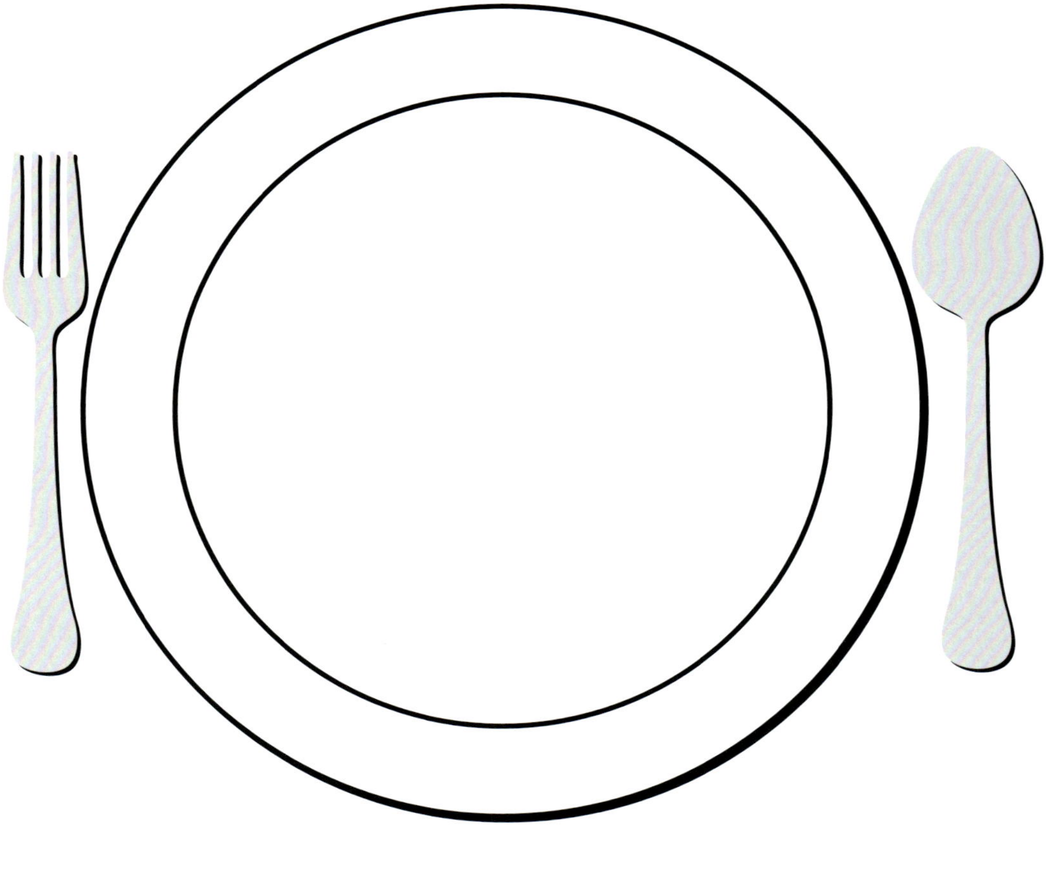

Write three words that describe your snack:

Yo soy todo Natural...
Y he creado un Yo sano.
Elijo de la naturaleza mis antojos y bocadillos,
como la manzana de un árbol!

Dibuja un bocadillo sano en tu plato.

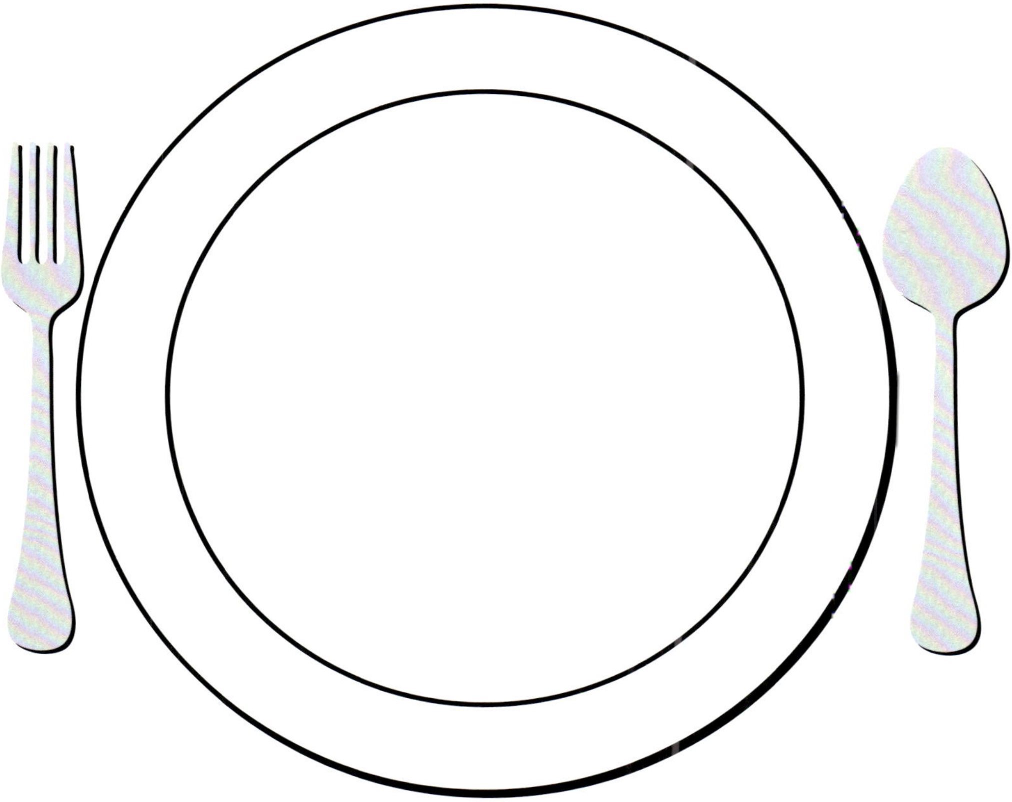

Escribe tres palabras que describan tu bocadillo:

____

____

____

I Am Alive!
So, I eat foods that are alive, too.
Like delicious fruits and veggies,
Which make me feel like new!

Read the names of the fruits and vegetables below. Write each word in the correct column on the chart.

Apples Oranges Broccoli Pears Carrots Cherries Grapes Green Beans Peas Cabbages Spinach Peaches

FRUITS	VEGETABLES

How many words can you make from the letters in "Fruits and Vegetables"?

Yo estoy Vivo!
Así que como alimentos vivos, también
Como las deliciosas frutas y vegetales,
Los cuales me hacen sentir como nuevo!

Lee los nombres de las frutas y verduras abajo. Escribe cada palabra en la columna correcta.

Manzana
Naranjas
Brócoli
Uvas
Ejotes
Duraznos
Zanahorias
Espinaca
Chicharos
Peras
Cerezas
Col

FRUTAS	VERDURAS

¿Cuantas palabras puedes formar usando las letras de las "frutas y las verduras"?

I Am Renewed!
By good things I eat and drink.
So very important, too, are
The good thoughts I choose to think.

I will frown.

I am healthy!

I will eat an apple.

I will watch TV.

I can choose my thoughts! Cross out the negative thoughts and practice reading aloud the positive ones!

I will eat candy.

I will play outside.

I can help.

I will smile.

Yo soy y me renuevo!
Por que las cosas buenas que como y bebo
Son tan importantes también, como los buenos
Pensamientos que elijo pensar.

Frunciré
el ceño

Yo soy sano!

Me comeré
una manzana

Mirare
televisión

Yo decido lo que pienso!
Tacho los pensamientos
negativos y practico recitar
en voz alta los positivos!

Comere dulces

Jugare afuera

Yo puedo
ayudar

Sonreire

I Am a Reader...
I read to learn what's good for me.
When it comes to good nutrition,
I take action! That's the key.

Scrambled Stories

The sentences below are not in the right order.
Number them in the correct sequence.

3 *He ate the sandwich.*
2 *He spread peanut butter on them.*
1 *He got out two slices of bread.*

______ *She built a nest.*
______ *Baby birds hatched from the eggs.*
______ *I saw a robin gathering twigs.*
______ *She laid four blue eggs.*

______ *I sneezed.*
______ *The pepper spilled out of the jar.*
______ *My nose began to itch.*

______ *She slid down the slide.*
______ *She climbed the ladder.*

Yo soy un buen lector...
Leo para aprender lo que es bueno para mi.
Cuando se trata de una buena nutrición,
Tomar acción! Es la clave!

Historias Revueltas

Las oraciones abajo no están en el orden correcto.
Numera en la secuencia correcta.

---

3 ______ *Él se comió el sándwich*

2 ______ *Él les unto la mantequilla de cacahuate*

1 ______ *Él sáco dos rebanadas de pan*

______ *Ella hizo un nido*

______ *los pajaritos salieron de sus huevos.*

______ *Vi a un pájaro petirrojo recogiendo ramas*

______ *Estornudé*

______ *La pimienta se derramo afuera del frasco.*

______ *Me dio comezón en la nariz*

______ *Ella se deslizó en el tobogán*

______ *Ella subió la escalera*

______ *Ella cayó sobre sus pies*

I Am Carefree!
When I let go of all concerns,
Like when I fly my kite,
My peace of mind returns.

"POP" the balloons by crossing out the letters that spell FEAR. What do the letters on the remaining balloons spell?

____

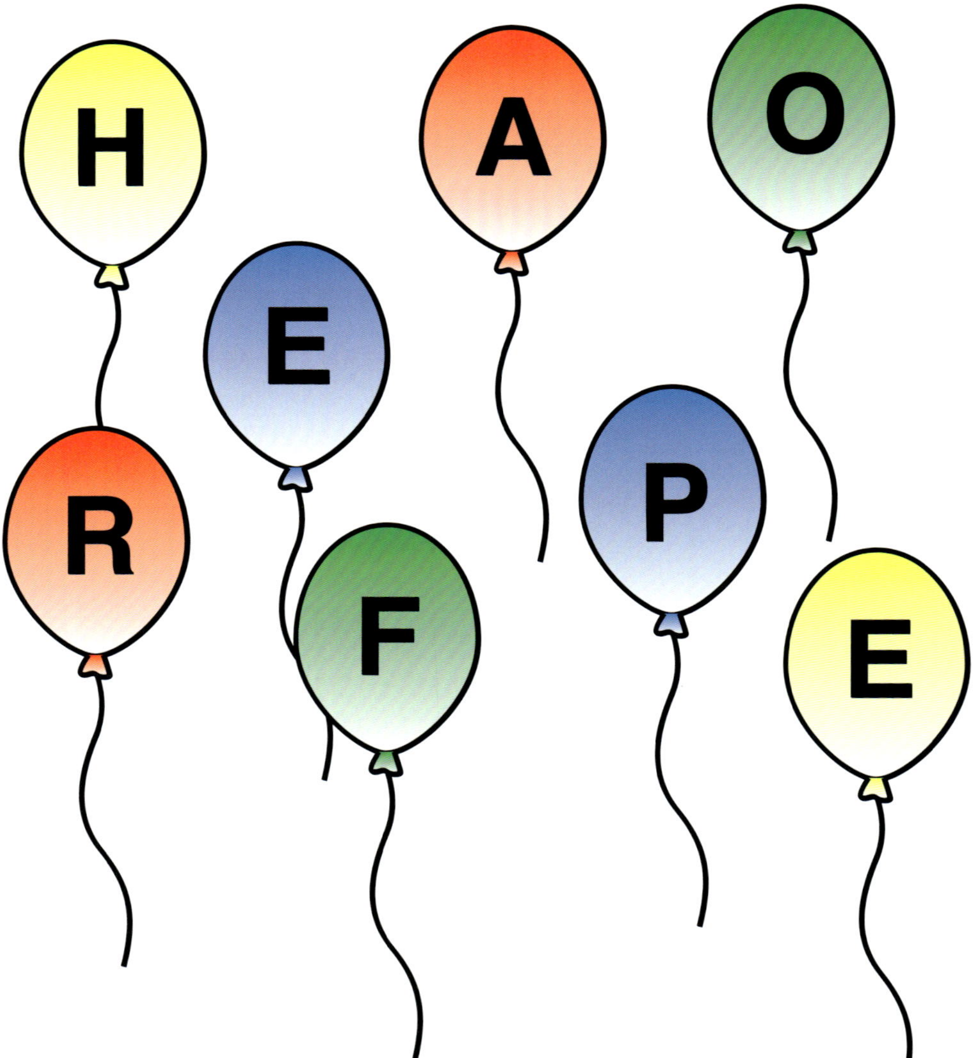

Yo Soy Despreocupado...
Cuando dejo atrás todas mis preocupaciones,
como cuando vuelo mi cometa,
mi paz mental regresa

"Truena" los globos tachando las letras que forman la palabra MIEDO. Como se deletrean las palabras que quedan?

____

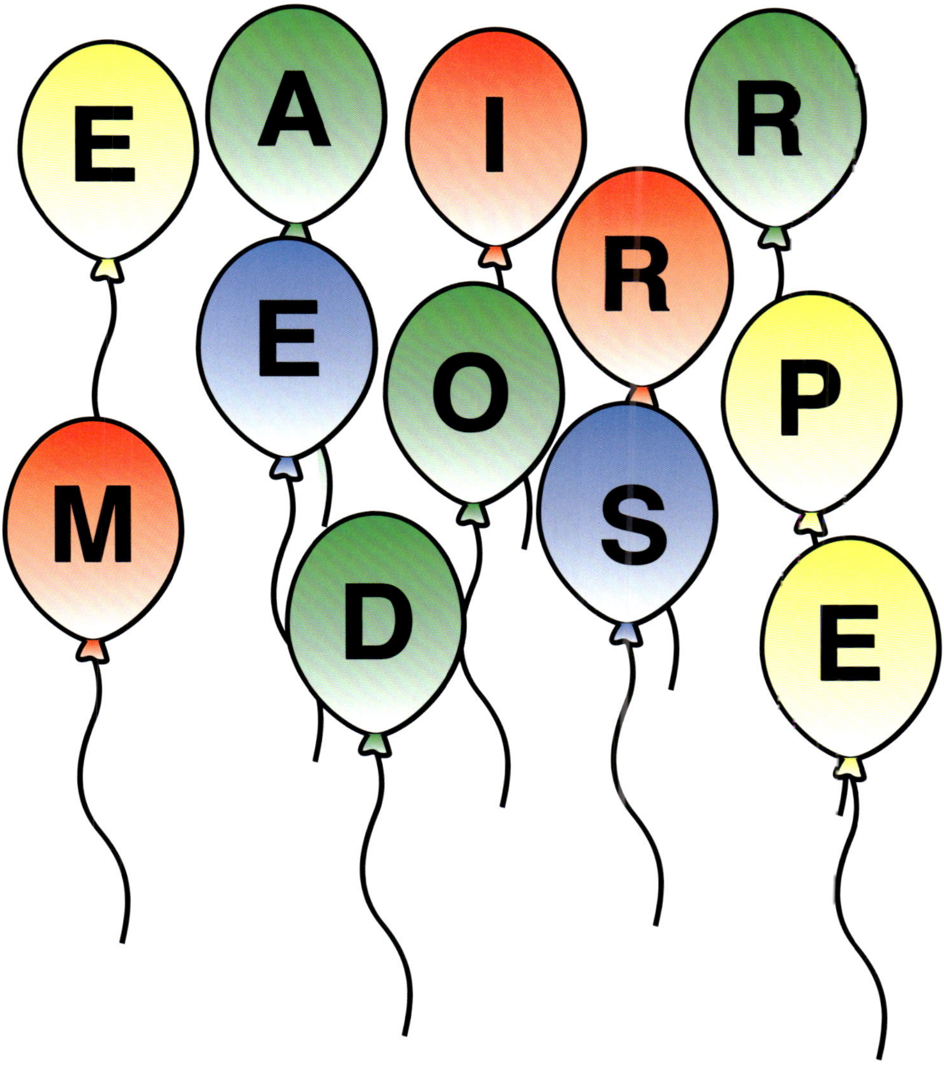

I Am Quiet!
When I take time for me,
I take time to be still,
And take a deep breath, or two, or three.

Quiet Time Bingo

Circle each activity you can do quietly for at least 10 minutes. Can you get 5 in a row?

____

Read a book	Watch birds flying	Look at the stars	Daydream	Count the leaves on a plant
Draw a picture	Sit quietly	Smell flowers	Write in my diary	Play with clay
Listen to the wind	Clean my room	**BONUS SQUARE**	Find a spiderweb	Make a daisy chain
Take a walk	Do a puzzle	Breathe slowly	Imagine you are a butterfly	Write a recipe
Look at the clouds	Lie on my bed	Listen to my heart-beat	Write a story	Blow bubbles

Yo Soy Tranquilo...
Cuando tomo tiempo para mí,
lo tomo para estar tranquilo.
Y respiro hondo una vez, o dos, o tres.

Tiempo
Bingo en Silencio

Haz un círculo en cada actividad que puedas hacer en silencio durante al menos 10 minutos.
¿Puedes poner 5 en una fila?

Lee un libro	Ve los pajaros volar	Mira las estrellas	Sueña despierto	Cuenta las hojitas de la planta
Haz un dibujo	Siéntate calladito	Huele las flores	Escribe en mi diario	Juega con plastilina
Escucha el viento	Limpia tu cuarto	**CASILLA BONO**	Encuentra una telaraña	Haz una cadena de margaritas
Toma un paseo	Haz un rompec-abezas	Respira despacio	Imagina que eres Mariposa	Escribe una receta
Mira las nubes	Recuestate en mi cama	Escucha mi corazón	Escribe una historia	Sopla burbujas

Singing Glasses

I Am Music!
Feeling the sounds inside my Soul.
I love to sing and dance,
Making me happy, joyful and whole.

Try making some singing glasses!

Fill some glasses partially with water, then rub a slightly wet finger tip around the rim and listen to the sounds you can make.

The more water you put in the glass, the deeper the note it will play.

Try tapping the rim of each glass with a pencil or spoon for another kind of sound!

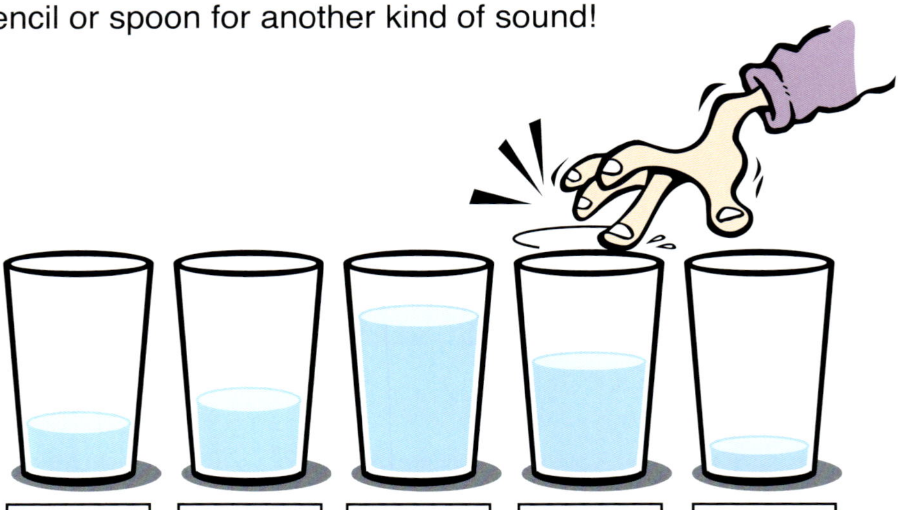

1/2	1/8	3/4	3/4	2/3
1/4	1/3	1/2	1/2	1/8

Under each glass, circle the fraction that best describes how much of the glass is filled with water.

Vasos que Cantan

Yo Soy Música!
Y siento todos los sonidos dentro de mi alma
Me encanta cantar y bailar,
Haciéndome feliz, alegre y completo

Haz cantar los vasos!

Llena los vasos parcialmente con agua, después rosa ligeramente la punta de tu dedo mojado alrededor y escucha los sonidos que se hacen.

Entre menos agua le pongas al vaso, el sonido de la nota será mas profundo

Prueba tocar la orilla del vaso con un lápiz o una cuchara para otro tipo de sonidos!

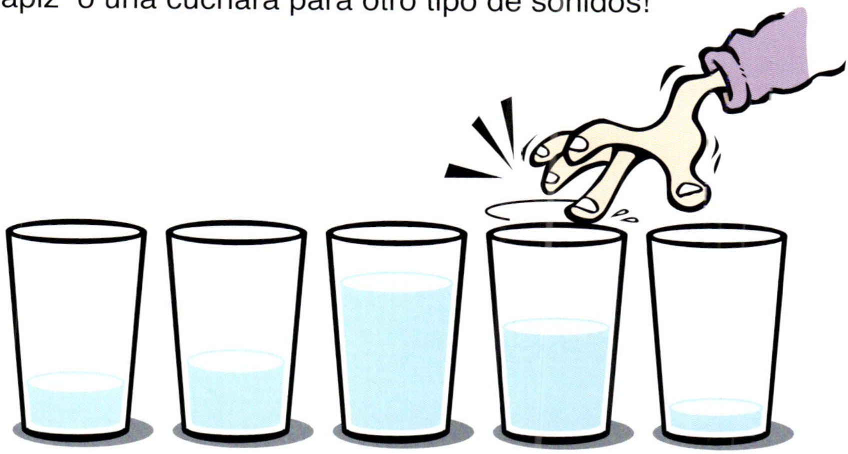

1/2	1/8	3/4	3/4	2/3
1/4	1/3	1/2	1/2	1/8

Bajo cada vaso, has un circulo en la fracción que mejor Describa la cantidad de agua que hay en el vaso.

I Am Laughter!
And what a joy it is to know,
That every time I laugh,
I feel good from head to toe.

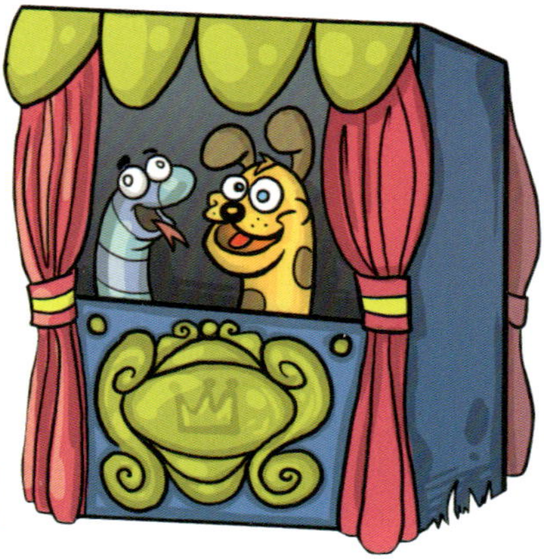

Laughter is good for you!

To discover the answer to each riddle, write the letter in the alphabet that comes before each letter under the line. Part of the first one is done for you.

What gets wetter the more it dries?	A / B _ / U O / P _ / X _ / F L / M
What goes up and down but never moves?	T U B J S T
What asks no questions, but demands an answer?	B Q I P O F
What do you call a camel at the North Pole?	M P T U

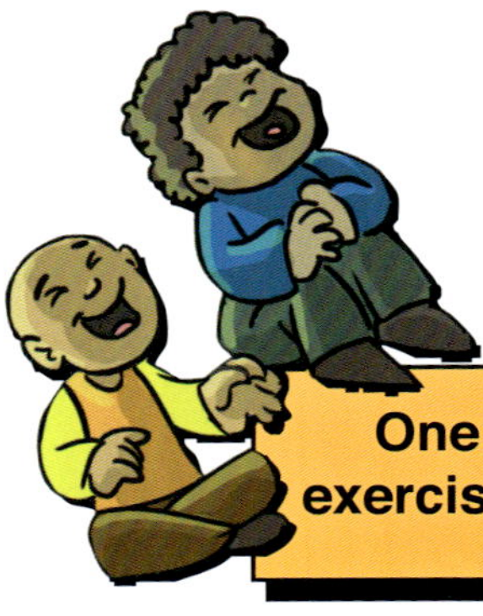

One hundred laughs is as much exercise as 15 minutes of bike riding!

Yo Soy la Risa!
Y que alegría es saber
que cada vez que río,
me siento bien de la cabeza a los pies.

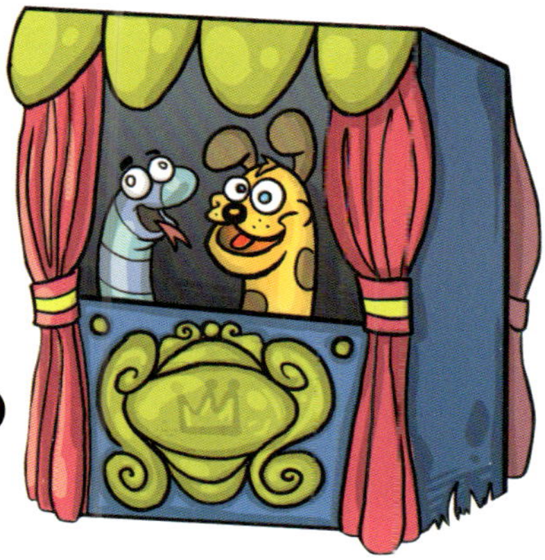

Reír es bueno para ti!

Para descubrir la respuesta de cada adivinanza, escribe la letra del alfabeto que esta antes de cada letra en la respuesta. La primera de ellas ya esta hecha para ti.

Que se moja mas cuando seca?

U _ _   _ O _ _ L _
V O B   U P B M M B

Que subre y baja pero nunca se mueve?

_ _ _ _ _ _ _ _ _
F T D B M F S B T

Quien hace preguntas pero no pide respuestas?

_ _
V O

_ _ _ _ _ _ _ _
U F M F G P O P

Como se le llama al Camello en el Polo Norte?

_ _ _ _ _ _ _
Q F S E J E P

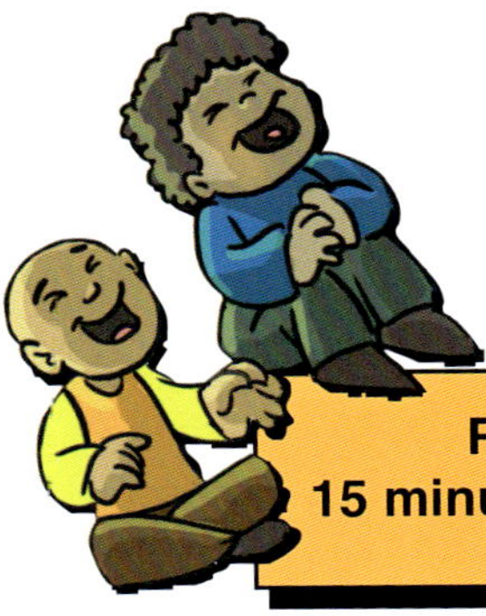

Reír cien veces equivale a 15 minutos de ejercicio en tu bicicleta!

I Am Playful...
And I do what makes me happy.
As long as it's good,
I'll be energized and snappy!

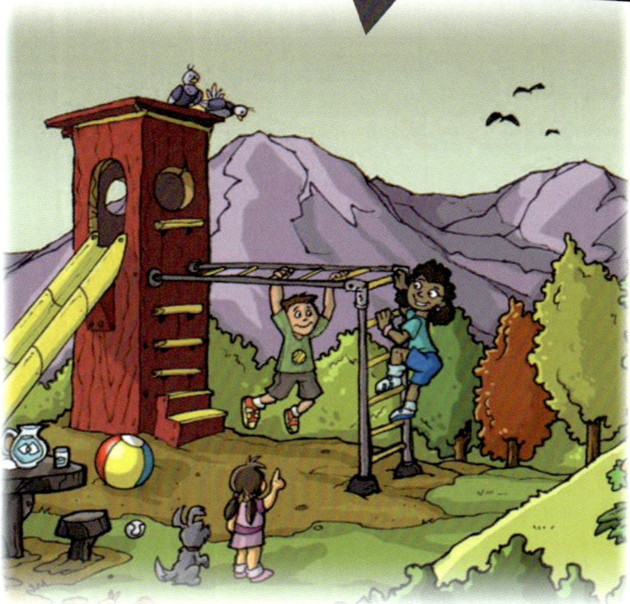

Can you find the 10 differences between these two images?

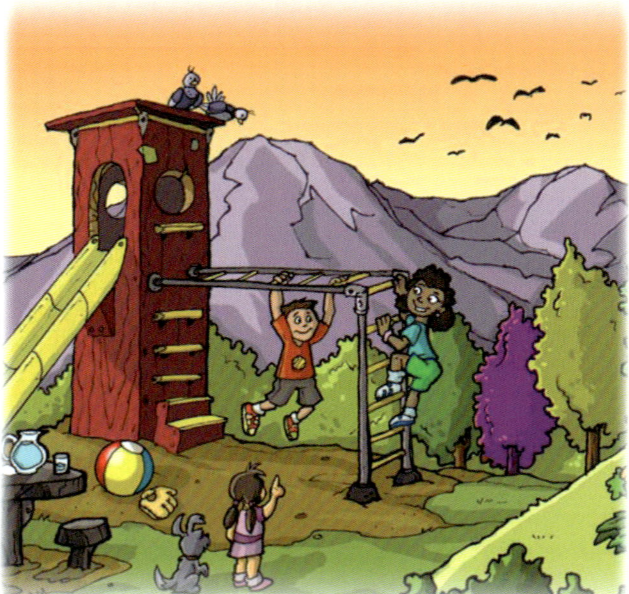

Yo Soy Juguetón!
Y hago lo que me hace feliz.
Mientras sea bueno,
me vigoriza y da energia

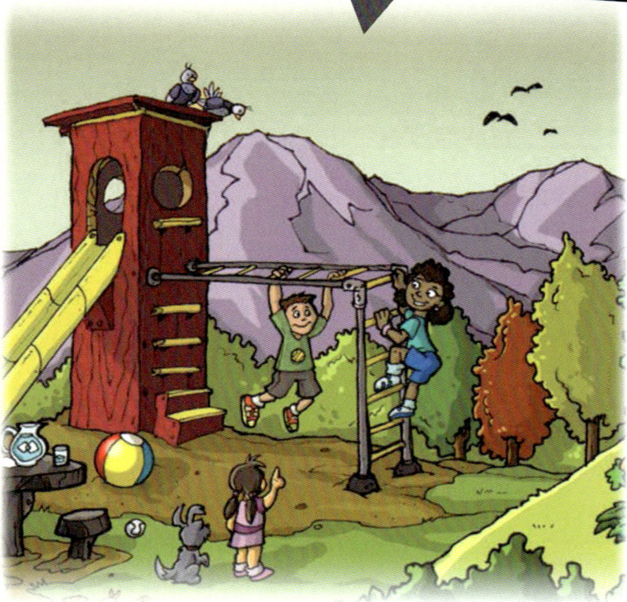

Puedes encontrar 10
cosas diferentes
En estos dibujos?

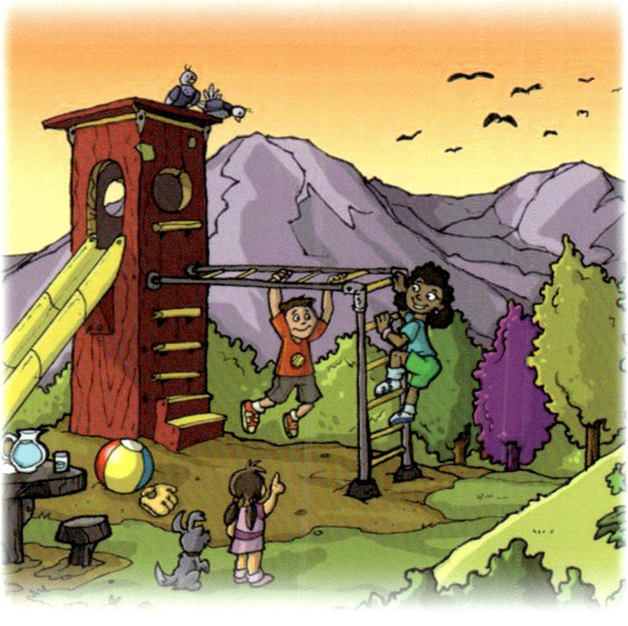

Now, I Am Healthy!
In each and every way,
Making the best choices,
Each and every day.

In the box below, write or draw two or more things that you do to be healthy.

Ahora, Yo Soy Sano!
En cada uno y todos los sentidos.
Tomando las mejores decisiones,
cada día y todos los días!

En el marco abajo, escribe
o dibuja dos o mas cosas de lo
que haces para mantenerte sano.

A Message from Steve and Marilyn About Making Healthy Choices

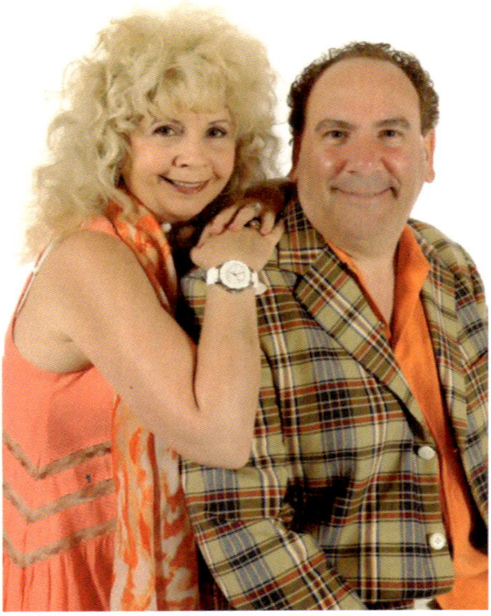

Health is our highest priority. As the greatest gift we can give ourselves, we can't take it for granted. And when our health is challenged, we feel the ripple effects in every aspect of our lives. That's why we need to expand our children's health awareness. Let's make it easier for our children to make more positive choices.

Steve wrote *I Am Healthy!* to inspire and motivate children to take actions that support their health and well-being. All children face choices, daily, that affect their health. Some of these choices may include:

- Breakfast: skipping? Or eating?
- Fitness: working on the computer, talking on the phone? Or going outside for fresh air and exercise?
- Transportation: riding in a car? Or walking? Riding a bike?
- Food: stuffing junk food? Or consuming nutritious food?
- Rest: staying up playing video games, or texting into all hours, and waking up exhausted? Or relaxing before bed and getting a full night's sleep?
- Fluids: drinking soda? Or hydrating with pure water?

This list comprises only a handful of choices that children face every day. Too often children find it easier to stay in unhealthy patterns than to change and make healthier choices. However, what are some of the benefits of making healthy choices?

- Feeling alive and alert
- Accessing focused attention
- Feeling good in your body
- Enjoying a healthy body and a sound mind

Our sincere hope? That *I Am Healthy!* supports our children to make the very best choices for their health. Why is their health so important? So children can share their talents and gifts to make dynamic differences in the world. They are our hope for a positive, sustainable future, and for a world that serves everyone.

— Steve Viglione and Dr. Marilyn Powers
Authors of The Love~Wisdom Series for Children and Adults
Co-Founders of The I AM Foundation

Un mensaje de Steve and Marilyn Tomando Decisiones Sanas

La salud es nuestra más alta prioridad. Es el regalo más grande que nos podemos dar a nosotros mismos, no lo podemos tomar a la ligera. Y cuando nuestra salud es amenazada, sentimos el efecto dominó que se propaga en cada aspecto de nuestras vidas. Es por eso que tenemos que extender la consciencia de salud en nuestros niños. Hagamos algo que facilite a nuestros niños tomar decisiones más positivas.

Steve escribió Yo Soy Sano! Para inspirar y motivar a los niños a tomar las acciones que apoyarán su salud y bienestar. Todos los niños enfrentan decisiones, diariamente, que afectan su salud. Algunas de estas decisiones pueden incluir:

- Desayuno: omitir ? O comer ?
- Ejercicio: trabajar en la computadora, hablar por teléfono? O ir afuera a tomar aire fresco y hacer ejercicio?
- Transporte: manejando en el auto? O caminando? Manejando bicicleta ?
- Comida: llenarse de comida chatarra? O Consumir alimentos nutritivos?
- Descanso: quedarse despierto jugando videojuegos, o mandando textos hasta altas horas de la noche, y despertar agotado? O relajarse antes de acostarse y ganar una noche completa?
- Líquidos: Tomar refrescos? O hidratarte con agua pura?

Esta lista incluye sólo un puñado de opciones que enfrentan los niños todos los días. Demasiado a menudo a los niños se les hace más fácil permanecer en patrones malsanos que cambiar y tomar decisiones más sanas. Sin embargo, Cuáles son algunos de los beneficios de hacer elecciones saludables?

- Sentirse vivo y alerta
- Acceder a una atención mas enfocada
- Sentirte bien en tu cuerpo
- Disfrutar de un cuerpo sano en una mente sana

Que esperamos sinceramente? ***Que Yo Soy Sano!*** apoye a nuestros hijos a tomar las mejores decisiones para su salud. Por que es tan importante su salud? Para que los niños puedan compartir sus talentos y dones mismos que los harán ser la diferencia en la dinámica del mundo. Ellos son nuestra esperanza para un futuro positivo y sostenible. Un mundo en servicio de todos.

~ Steve Viglione and Dr. Marilyn Powers
Autores de las Series Amor~Sabiduría para niños y adultos
Co-Fundadores de la Fundación YO SOY. (I AM Foundation)

A Message to Teachers from Vicki Whiting, Educator and Publisher of Kid Scoop®

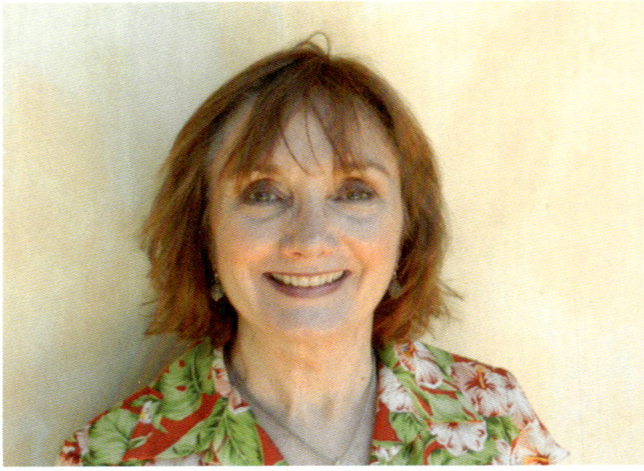

The ***I Am Healthy!*** book for children provides extraordinary opportunities for teachers to reinforce positive life choices and character education easily and effectively in the classroom. Students making healthy choices soon become alert, focused, and ready-to-learn. A healthy classroom with a caring atmosphere helps students feel safe. They feel better about themselves and more likely treat others with kindness and respect.

I was honored when Steve Viglione and Dr. Marilyn Powers of **The I AM Foundation** asked me to create workbook pages for their stunning book ***I Am Healthy! Affirmations for Health and Well-Being***. As a teacher, I know that mastery of any skill requires practice, practice, and more practice. And the more we make practicing skills playful, the more children find the repetition fun and effortless.

The ***I Am Healthy!*** book provides a valuable addition to the elementary school classroom. Beautiful illustrations and engaging poems draw the children in, as changing their choices sounds playful and engaging. The readers find the rhymes fun to read over and over, and easily memorized. The activities included in the ***Healthy Scoop*** pages easily and effortlessly commit the ***I Am Healthy!*** affirmations to a child's memory, thus internalizing key healthy-lifestyle choices.

Children internalize these affirmations and concepts, through repetition and memorization, thus impacting the choices they make about what they eat, how they exercise, and how they talk to others and themselves. Creating a positive atmosphere in the classroom enhances each child's ability to learn and grow into a caring and confident individual.

— Vicki Whiting, Educator
Publisher of Kid Scoop®
www.kidscoop.com

Un Mensaje a los Profesores de Vicki Whiting Educador y Editor de Kid Scoop®

El libro para niños **¡Yo Soy Sano!** ofrece oportunidades extraordinarias a los maestros para reforzar las opciones de vida positivas y formación de carácter fácilmente y eficazmente en el salón de clases. Los estudiantes que toman decisiones sanas demuestran estar alertas, enfocados y listos para aprender. Un salón de clases con una atmósfera cuidada ayuda a los estudiantes a sentirse seguros. Ellos se sienten mejor sobre sí mismos y lo más probable es que tratarán a los demás con amabilidad y respeto.

Para mi fue un honor que Steve Viglione y la Dra. Marilyn Powers de **La Fundacion Yo Soy** me pidieran crear las paginas de sus libros **¡Yo Soy Sano!** ***Afirmaciones para la Salud y Bienestar.*** Como educadora, yo sé que el dominio de cualquier habilidad requiere práctica, práctica y más practica. Y entre mas hagamos estas estas habilidades divertidas, aún más los niños disfrutarán la repetición de aprender sin esfuerzo.

El libro **¡Yo Soy Sano!** Proporciona una valiosa adición a los salones de clases en las escuelas primarias. Bellas ilustraciones y simpáticos poemas atraen a los niños, mientras van cambiando sus opciones de una forma mas divertida y atractiva. Nuestros pequeños lectores encontrarán las rimas divertidas de leer una y otra y otra vez, fácil de memorizar. Las actividades incluidas en las paginas de ***Scoop de la salud*** fácilmente y sin esfuerzo crean un compromiso de afirmación **¡Yo Soy Sano!** en la memoria de los niños, Y así internalizan la clave para optar por un estilo de vida más saludable.

Los niños internalizan estas afirmaciones y conceptos, a través de la repetición y memorización, al mismo tiempo que impactan las decisiones que hacen acerca de lo que comen, como se ejercitan, y su forma de hablar con otros y ellos mismos. Creando una atmósfera positiva en los salones de clases mejorará la capacidad de cada niño de aprender, crecer y convertirse en una persona cariñosa y segura.

Vicki Whiting, Educator
Editor del Kid Scoop®
www.kidscoop.com

A Message to Parents and Teachers, from Christopher Oscar, Father of Two

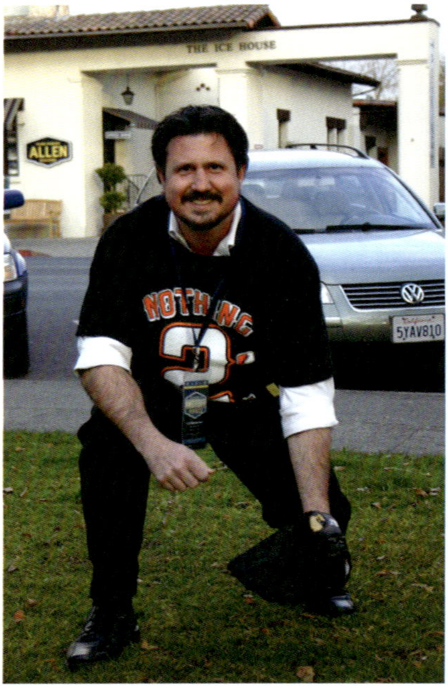

As a parent of two young children, I see, firsthand, how unhealthy foods affect behaviors in negative ways. I also notice how wholesome, organic foods with a healthy dose of spring water bring beautiful glows to my children's faces.

Do we spend time reading labels? You bet we do! However, what ends up on children's plates is not always easy to control. Birthday parties, Halloween, and Valentine's Day tremendously pressure children to eat junk food.

Many parents don't understand the relationship between feeling good, being healthy, and what kids eat and drink. The good news? My children understand. I talked to my children about the effects of sugar and how it alters their mood and ultimately their health. I encourage all parents and teachers to discuss this with their children and their students.

What about exercise and reading, versus watching TV or playing video games? Once a child turns off the TV and engages in drawing, reading, or playing outside, a whole, new child seems to emerge!

I am so grateful for Steve Viglione and Dr. Marilyn Powers for writing *I Am Healthy! Affirmations for Health and Well-Being* for our children. We are the ones entrusted with keeping our children healthy and safe and encouraging them to live to their fullest potential. *I Am Healthy!* brings to light many different aspects of health for children and parents to focus upon—eating live foods filled with nutrients the body needs, drinking water, exercising, playing with good friends, enjoying nature, and more.

Christopher Oscar
Father and Realtor at Frank Howard Allen Realtors, Sonoma, CA
http://www.yoursonoma.com

Mensaje para Padres y Maestros de parte de Christopher Oscar, Padre de Dos

Como padre de dos niños pequeños, Veo de primera mano, como los alimentos malsanos afectan su comportamiento en forma negativa. También me doy cuenta cómo los alimentos completos y orgánicos con una buena dosis de agua de manantial trae un resplandor de belleza a las caras de mis hijos.

Que si me tomo el tiempo de leer etiquetas? Se lo apuesto. Sin embargo lo que usted pone en el plato de su hijo no siempre es fácil de controlar. Las fiestas de cumpleaños, La noche de brujas, El día de San Valentín presionan tremendamente a los niños a consumir comida chatarra.

Muchos padres no entienden la relación entre sentirse bien, a estar sano, y lo que los niños comen y beben. La buena noticia es que mis hijos entienden. Les he hablado de los efectos del azúcar y como altera su estado de animo y principalmente su salud. Invito a todos los padres y maestros a hablar de esto con sus hijos y sus estudiantes.

Que tal ejercicio y lectura, en vez de ver televisión y video juegos? Una vez que el niño apaga la televisión y elabora un dibujo, lee o sale a jugar, emerge un niño nuevo.

Estoy muy agradecido con Steve Viglione y la Dr. Marilyn Powers por haber creado estas series de libros dedicados a iluminar a los niños y a sus padres sobre hábitos saludables. Comer alimentos vivos llenos de nutrientes que el cuerpo necesita, agua potable, ejercicio, jugar con los amigos, disfrutar de la naturaleza y más.

Christopher Oscar
Padre y Agente Inmobiliario en Frank Howard Allen Realtors,
Sonoma, CA.
http://www.yoursonoma.com

A Message to the Parents and Teachers from Carole Peccorini, RN, MA

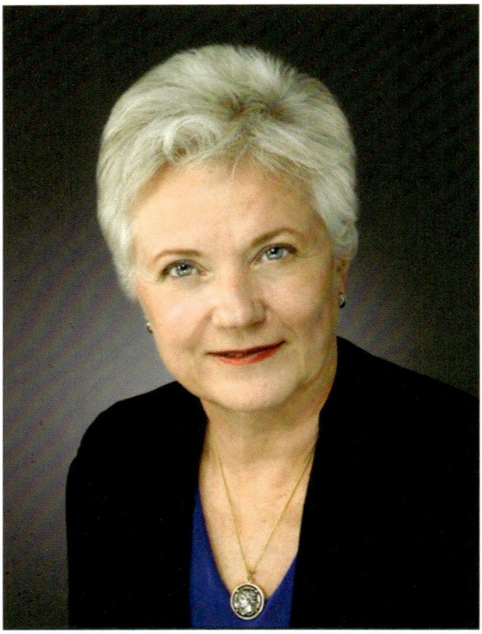

I Am Healthy! Affirmations for Health and Well-Being helps our children be more sensitive and aware of making choices that keep them healthy and safe.

Is the Universe a friendly place? Albert Einstein says our answer to this question determines everything about what we believe and experience in our lives. How do we teach our children about safety as a core health practice without over-stimulating fears of an unfriendly world? I think of past generations of parents and teachers who explored answers to this question.

While modern-day risks include cars, traffic, and other possible scenarios, earlier generations feared the forest and wild animals. Imagine parents or elders teaching their young about the forest and what to do if lost in that forest. Where is the food, the hidden sources of water and shelter? What about preying animals? What do today's children need to know about respecting fire? How about plants and food that nourish, heal, or cause illness? What about seeking safety during earthquakes, violent weather, or stormy seas? Why drink water on a hot day while playing soccer?

I Am Healthy! Affirmations for Health and Well-Being expresses how our children exist as part of this matrix of life and helps guide them in ways that strengthen them. An affirmation for safety and health: "I am aware of my world, and I make safe and healthy choices."

Carole Peccorini, RN, MA
Big Ideas and Rich Conversations with Women
http://sonomabigideas.blogspot.com

Un Mensaje para los Padres y Maestros de parte de Carole Peccorini

Yo Soy sano! Afirmaciones para la salud y el bienestar ayuda a nuestros hijos a ser más sensibles y conscientes en las decisiones que eligen para mantenerse sanos y seguros.

Es el Universo un lugar amistoso? Albert Einstein dice que nuestra respuesta a esta pregunta determina todo sobre lo que creemos y experimentamos en nuestras vidas.

¿Cómo les enseñamos a nuestros hijos acerca de la seguridad como núcleo de una práctica de salud sin sobre-estimular sus miedos en un mundo poco amigable? Esto me hace pensar en generaciones pasadas de padres y maestros que exploraron respuestas a estas preguntas.

Mientras que hoy en día los riesgos incluyen automóviles, tráfico y otros posibles escenarios, las generaciones anteriores le temían a los bosques y animales salvajes. Imagínese a los padres o ancianos enseñando a sus jóvenes acerca de los bosques y que hacer si se perdieran en ese bosque. ¿Dónde está la comida, las fuentes ocultas de agua y la vivienda? ¿Y que paso con animales de presa? ¿Qué es lo que los niños de hoy necesitan saber sobre respetar el fuego? ¿Qué pasa con las plantas y los alimentos que nutren, curan, o causan la enfermedad? ¿ y la busca de seguridad durante terremotos, climas violentos, o mares tempestuosos?
¿Por qué beber agua en un día caluroso mientras juegas fútbol?

Yo Soy sano! Afirmaciones para la salud y el bienestar expresa cómo nuestros niños existen como parte de esta matriz de la vida y ayuda a guiarlos de una manera que los fortalece. Una afirmación para la seguridad y la salud es: " Yo soy consciente de mi mundo, y tomo decisiones seguras y saludables "

Carole Peccorini RN, MA.
Buenas ideas y Ricas Conversaciones entre Mujeres
http://sonomabigideas.blogspot.com

The I AM Foundation's
Buy-One, Gift-One Program

"Whenever you purchase a Love~Wisdom Series™ book, another book is gifted to a child somewhere in the world."

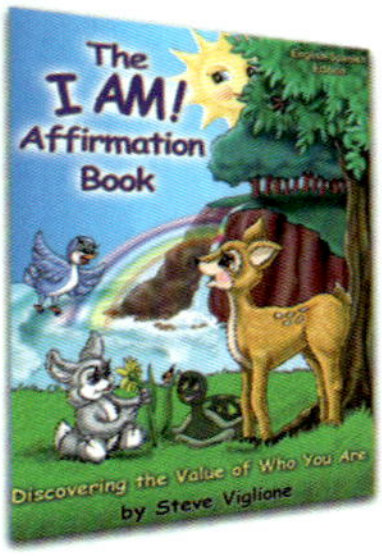

The I AM! Affirmation Book and Curriculum
Discovering the Value of Who You Are
By Steve Viglione
For pre-K through 4th grade

I Am The Earth and Curriculum
Positive Affirmations for Loving Our Planet
By Steve Viglione
For pre-K through 6th grade

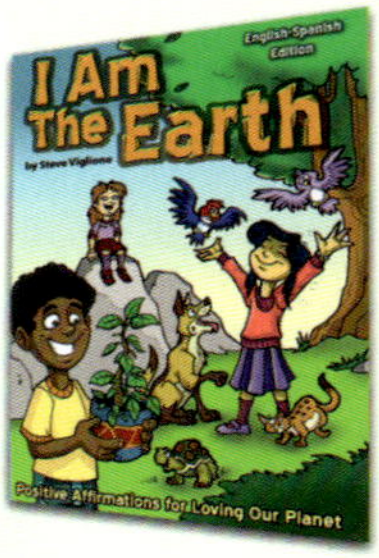

The I AM! Affirmation Book For Teens and Young Adults
Empowering Who You Are
By Steve Viglione

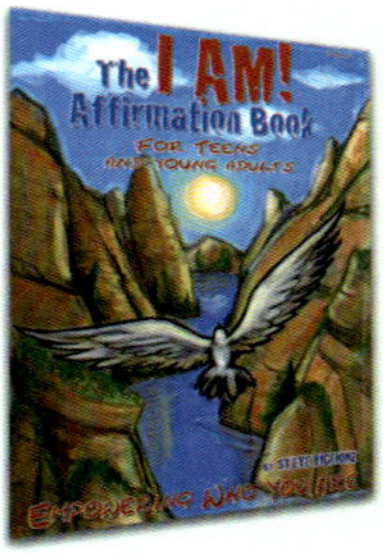

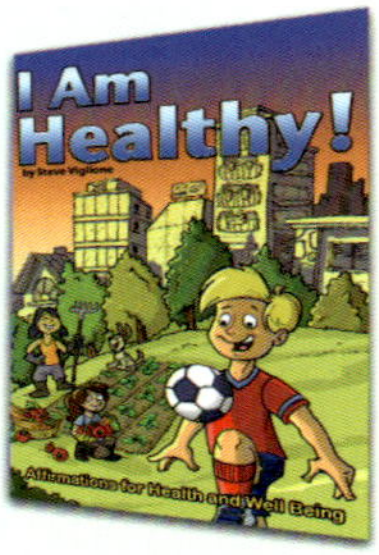

I Am Healthy!
Affirmations for Health and Well-Being
By Steve Viglione
For pre-K through 6th grade

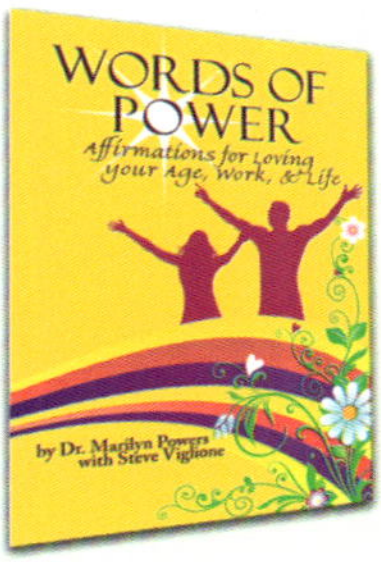

Words of Power
Affirmations for Loving your Age, Work & Life
By Dr. Marilyn Powers
An empowering guide for adults

The Bridge and Companion Workbook
A Seven-Stage Map to Redefine Your Life and Purpose
By Dr. Marilyn Powers
For adults moving through change and transition

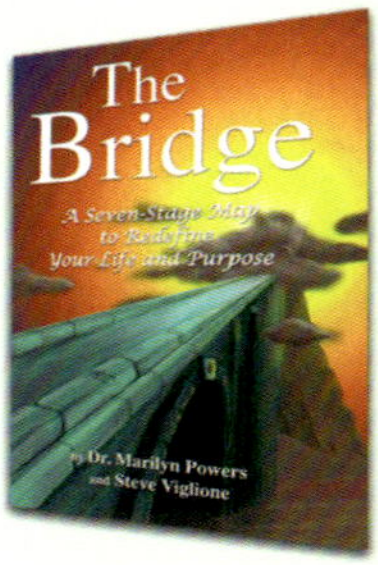

Make a profound impact by ordering books or making a donation to support our programs at
www.iamfoundation.org
or call 619.297.7010

Follow Us On:

Books available at Amazon.com
eBooks available on Kindle, iTunes, Nook, Reader and Smashwords.com

The Power of Christian Mediation

Developing Spirit Led Outcomes

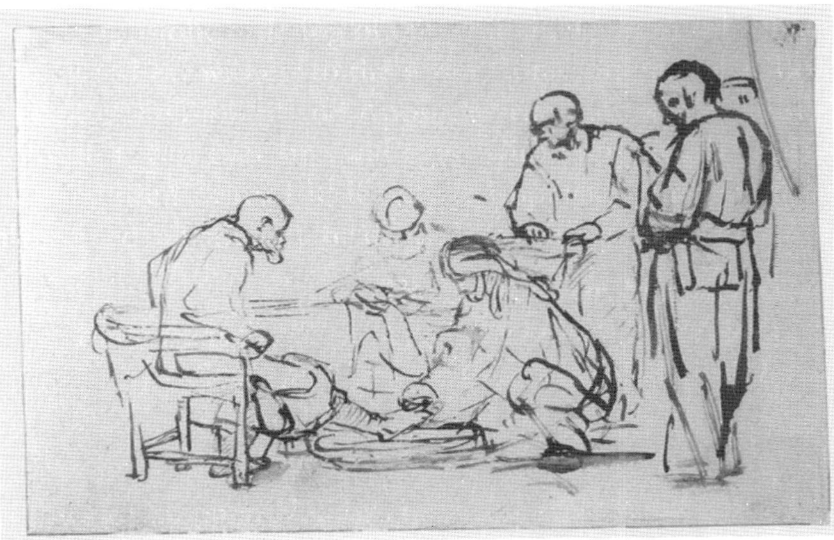

Bishop Trevor Walters

Foreword by Archbishop Foley Beach

Anglican Liturgy Press

Published by Anglican House Publishers® registered trade name of Anglican House Media Ministry, Inc., Newport Beach, California. You can find us at *anglicanhousepublishers.org*. Text set in Baskerville typeface. Printed by Asia Printing Co., Ltd., Seoul, Korea.

Anglican Liturgy Press

Second Printing 2020

ISBN 978-0-9993010-8-2

About the Cover Art

Rembrandt's Drawings include dozens of Christian subjects, including this one c. 1655. It depicts Christ washing his Disciples' feet. The message of scripture is clear enough: "If I then, your Lord and Teacher, have washed your feet, you also ought to wash one another's feet." (John 13:14)

The artist's scene, showing as it does several figures, seems appropriate to Christian Mediation, inasmuch as while there may be but two or more disputants, there are always bystanders involved to one extent or another. They too will be blessed as they observe the outcome of Christian Mediation, with the principals submitting to one another out of reverence for Christ. (Ephesians 5:21)

Dedication

This book is dedicated to the men and women who regularly risk their health and reputation when stepping between warring parties. I salute peacemakers everywhere who see peace as not just the absence of conflict but instead the re-establishment of trust and respect.

In particular this dedication goes to my wife Dede who has always been a peacemaker, whom I trust with all my heart and respect with all my being.

A Mediator's Prayer

(A Prayer of Saint Francis)

Lord, make me an instrument of your peace.
Where there is hatred, let me sow love.
Where there is injury, pardon.
Where there is doubt, faith.
Where there is despair, hope.
Where there is darkness, light.
Where there is sadness, joy.

O Divine Master, grant that I may not so much seek
To be consoled, as to console;
To be understood, as to understand;
To be loved, as to love.
For it is in giving that we receive.
It is in pardoning that we are pardoned,
And it is in dying that we are born to Eternal Life.
Amen.

Contents

Contents

Foreword

Our Lord Jesus Christ calls his followers to love one another (John 13:35). He also discusses the importance of forgiving one another (Matthew 6:12, 14).

The Apostle Paul further developed this emphasis in the New Testament Church when he wrote to the believers in Colossae:

> "Put on then, as God's chosen ones, holy and beloved, compassionate hearts, kindness, humility, meekness, and patience, bearing with one another and if one has a complaint against another, forgiving each other; as the Lord has forgiven you, so you must also forgive." (Colossians 3:12,13)

He wrote the believers in the church at Philippi:

> "I entreat Euodia and I entreat Synche to agree in the Lord. Yes, I ask you also, true companion, help these women, who have labored side by side with me in the gospel together with Clement and the rest of my fellow workers, who names are in the book of life." (Philippians 4:2,3)

To the believers in the church at Ephesus he is even more direct:

> "Do not grieve the Holy Spirit of God, by whom you were sealed for the day of redemption. Let all bitterness and wrath and anger and clamor and slander be put away from you, along with all malice. Be kind to one another,

> tenderhearted, forgiving one another, as God in Christ forgave you." (Ephesians 4:29-32)

As in the days of the New Testament, the human condition calls us to confront one another in love and forgiveness from a mind being renewed and transformed by the Holy Spirit (Romans 12:1,2)—living in peace with our brothers and sisters in the Lord. And yet, we see division and disharmony among followers of Jesus in too many church bodies and congregations, and in too many personal and family relationships. So often, good and generous people get at odds with one another and come to an impasse unable to reconcile their differences.

Sometimes these conflicts are based on their different interpretations of the Bible, their personality differences, wounding and mean behaviors, or a refusal to walk in the Holy Spirit (Galatians 5:16-23). However, all division and broken relationships have restorative possibilities because of the Cross of Jesus Christ and the Presence of the Holy Spirit. The exhortations by Jesus and the Apostle Paul for Christ-followers to love one another and to forgive one another demonstrate that this is a possibility, or else they would not have asked us to do this.

Bishop Trevor Walters' insights and long experience are remarkable in helping faithful followers of Jesus, and those in the corporate world and marketplace, to resolve seemingly impossible barriers between them. Bishop Walters understands not only the Biblical precepts concerning reconciliation, but his wisdom in the realm of human behavior has much to offer too.

Although I am hesitant to use the word mediation because of the misuse and misapplication of the word, Bishop Walters understands mediation and his guidance will help bring reconciliation in impossible situations. Read what he has written. Reflect on it and read it again. And then put this into practice in your life and ministry, loving and forgiving one another in Christ.

The Most Rev. Dr. Foley Beach
Archbishop and Primate, Anglican Church in North America
Bishop, Anglican Diocese of the South

Introduction

Church conflict is epidemic with splits within denominations, division in local churches, conflicts among pastors and congregations, and more. Even some bishops and pastors war with one another. And of course families are impacted with husbands, wives and children sometimes divided.

This book is written for those who have a deep love for the Church, and yet lack a road map for resolution when dealing with conflict. We will need a veritable army of peacemakers if Jesus' High Priestley prayer, "that they may be one" would be fulfilled in our generation.

Conflict is a spiritual stronghold that can immobilize even the strongest spiritual leaders, as we will review in greater detail. Given the amount of fear and helplessness with which church leaders approach conflict, one would think the Bible is silent on the subject. It is not so at all, as we'll see in this book.

Sadly, the secular world has noticed the church's failure to be a mediating force and stepped in to provide a mediation road map. My own training as a Circuit Civil Mediator with Florida's Supreme Court was one of the most invigorating educational experiences I ever had. That secular course gave me new insights into the great heritage of the Bible concerning mediation. I will attempt to provide a "vision for conflict" to empower those who must deal with conflict almost daily. After years of stepping into other peoples' disasters, I have acquired a quiet confidence that, when followed, the principles outlined in this book will bring resolution to conflict. Conflict that has reigned and ruled for perhaps years can be actually gone for good!

My Christian mediation strategies were first developed in theory when I was a university lecturer. Then as a priest I was "baptized" in the River of Church Conflicts, and thereafter "confirmed" in the wrenching conflict between the Anglican Mission in America and the Anglican Church of North America (ACNA). Here and there I have mediated conflict in multiple Orthodox groups, both within and outside the Church of England.

Trained mediators have a valuable set of tools in their toolbox to help them resolve tough issues. We will examine the basics and share some less than obvious approaches and techniques that can help untie the most stubborn knots one encounters in the mediation process.

My dear friend Canon Phil Ashey and were envisioning a course of training for mediators who could be deployed within ACNA. We had hoped to have two or more candidates from every Diocese attend a weekend course and become mediator apprentices. But we needed a textbook for this bold venture in Christian mediation. This is that textbook.

I had drafted the curriculum and was honored when top mediators heard of the project and wanted to be a part of the weekend. I simply told them that they could not come unless they were willing to present on a topic related to mediation. Having extracted their agreement to present at the first Christian Mediation weekend course in Atlanta in January 2017, I added one another stipulation: that they submit their presentations for inclusion in this book.

They all agreed. (This was one of the nicest results I ever negotiated!)

What a delight to have such outstanding contributors to this book.

Bishop Trevor Walters
Epiphany 2018

One

A Vision for Mediation

By Bishop Trevor Walters

Why the need for Christian mediation? Mediation is just mediation unless you mean mediation performed by a person with Christian beliefs. It is true that mediation and Christian mediation do have similar characteristics. One in particular is that for a mediation to be successful something must change hands. In the case of secular mediation, money is handed over and both parties leave resolved and unhappy that they did not get as much or, conversely, gave too much money to the other side. Do you really mean unhappy? If the mediation was considered successful then both parties involved resolved the problem. Plus it saved discovery costs and prevented a prolonged battle. Still, holding onto my thesis of unhappy, secular mediation works in a climate where there is little good will and both parties are concerned principally with their own needs. One or both parties suspect the other has provided financial statements or facts that misrepresent the actual facts. In some instances the information provided might be outright lies. So yes, relief that it is over without spending a major amount of money on legal fees, but an undercurrent exists that says, "It was not fair!" If you were still concerned with an aspect of the settlement years later, I'd say you were unhappy. The enduring long-term fruit of unhappiness is often resentment.

So, what would make one happy in Christian mediation? There is generally little or no money available in any church that I know to actually exchange hands. Indeed, if a church came in over budget and they were willing to pay money for mediation that deals with principle or doctrine, they would no doubt be unhappy with the outcome of compromised principles and doctrine.

For a mediation to be successful something must exchange hands. If no money is exchanged, then what better can be exchanged than repentance and forgiveness?

CHRISTIAN MEDIATION

What I have witnessed in Christian mediations is both parties leave with the issue resolved and are deeply happy to be back in Christian relationship. The resentment often seen at the end of secular mediation has been replaced by forgiveness resulting in a deeper lasting reconciliation.

Is this not one of the theories of the atonement: a divine exchange passing between hands? Atonement is achieved when a third party pays the price of the crime. The debt is settled, justice is done, and peace is achieved. As Paul writes in his letter to the Romans, "…while we were still sinners Christ died for us." (Roman 5:8) The divine peacemaker reconciles the world to himself and he immediately calls us to be reconcilers and peacemakers.

In the Beatitudes, the way of 'being with attitude', peacemakers are called blessed and they inherit the world. Christian mediators are following in the Father's footsteps and are called to function as the Father did through his agent, his son Jesus.

THE FIRST BIBLICAL MEDIATION

Let's explore the principle of the Great Grace Exchange. In the Old Testament book of Genesis, Chapters 31-34, secular mediation and Christian mediation are at war within Jacob. Lets look back to get the punch that comes in Genesis 33:4. Two brothers, Jacob and Esau, were born to Isaac. Jacob the younger brother would not by law get his fathers blessing and consequently would not receive an inheritance. The boy's mother Rebekah had a favorite son, and you guessed it. It was not Esau, the oldest. Mother and younger son schemed to cheat Esau out of his rightful inheritance. Suffice it to say they pulled it off, but it sent Jacob running for fear of a violent reprisal from Esau. Jacob was a fugitive for years, but his broken relationship with his brother was killing him on the inside. He decided to go to find his brother in the hope of reconciling.

How was he going to mediate the brokenness of the relationship? Let's be honest, the relationship was broken because Jacob deceived his brother. Jacob was now saying "I'll buy him off! I have lots of assets and I will gladly exchange half my cattle for a restored relationship with Esau." Jacob created an elaborate plan to get his servants to go ahead of him with successive gift packages aimed at breaking down Esau's supposed desire for revenge.

At this point Jacob was ready to start the mediation, and it was set for the next day at noon. Jacob must have had a rock for a pillow, because he had a very poor night's sleep. But he was not fighting a pillow; he was wrestling with a man. I don't know when he realized that the man represented God, but it happened. His desire for a real blessing also got him in the gut. So Jacob said to the man, "I will not let you go unless you bless me!" (Genesis 32:26b) Herein lies the basis for civil mediation: How much money will it take to appease my brother?

Good news for Jacob. He got the blessing from God, but because Jacob struggled with the man, God touched his hip and Jacob walked with a limp for the rest of his life. The hand of God had touched deep inside of Jacob. He was reconciled with God and that was essential as the vertical component of the mediation. Now he had to deal with his brother, who hated him. Jacob's worst fear was birthed as He saw Esau coming with 400 men. Jacob assumed the worst. After all, he had lived in a dark room for years, which is good for developing negative thoughts!

Jacob went ahead of all his entourage and bowed down seven times to the ground before Esau. But while Jacob was consumed with humility and repentant gestures he failed to see that his brother was running towards him and weeping. The Bible says Esau fell on Jacob's neck and kissed him. After numerous introductions, Esau asked Jacob to explain the meaning of the excessive gifts Jacob had offered him. The answer was poignant: "To find favor in your eyes, my Lord." (Geneses 33:8b)

Conditional acceptance is the name of this sad game. I can earn your love. Here is a great foreshadowing of the Gospel message that although we are cheating, deceiving, and lying people, we are granted unmerited favor by the one we hurt.

Esau trumpets grace by saying: "I already have plenty my brother. Keep what you have for yourself."(Genesis 33:9) Esau named Jacob as his brother, a big step toward healing their broken relationship. The relationship is further restored by Esau's forgiveness and Jacob's repentance. The grand exchange is complete and money played no part in the mediation.

Now that the relationship is healed, gifts are given by Jacob and received by Esau, but now they represent thank offerings rather than bribes. Jacob's own words to his brother speak so eloquently, "Please accept my blessing that is brought to you, because God has dealt graciously with me, and because I have enough." (Genesis 33:11)

In the encounter of Jacob and Esau, we see a basis for Christian mediation that is distinct from civil mediation.

Two striking differences emerge. First, the tokens or elements used to mediate are repentance and forgiveness. Second, the end goal is a restored relationship.

My limited experience as a civil mediator is that the end goal is to deal with a specific issue rather than the health of a relationship. The dominant restorative factor is money.

Rarely will an astute mediator recognize that for example, a patient or a motorist at the end of the day wants the doctor or driver to admit they made a mistake. It is typical that lawyers will counsel their clients against admission of liability. So a mediator who sees what is truly needed will often have their hands tied by representatives of our litigious world.

It is important to say how effective mediation is within the limits imposed upon it. When I certified as a Civil Mediator in 2010, with the Florida Supreme Court, all civil disputes had to first go to mediation. In 60% of the cases mediation successfully resolved the issue. Lest you think I have it in for mediators and mediation, I assure you it is exactly the opposite. I have never enjoyed a course more or been more inspired by seeing Florida mediators at work. I am deeply indebted to the Florida Supreme Court for allowing non-lawyers to become Circuit Court Civil Mediators. There were 34 in the course that year in Tampa, with only three non-lawyers.

The lawyers in the class were rightly suspicious of us and gave us some of the most complicated cases imaginable, in endless role-playing activities. Toward the end of the course one lawyer announced that the hazing was over when he said, "We lawyers were trained for win-lose, you only know win-win. We were trained to think inside the legal box, but you don't even know there is a box. Consequently, your solutions were very creative. Reluctantly, we admit you are good at this."

It is interesting to note that when a lawyer makes the shift to a win-win strategy they become fine mediators. I was talking to a lawyer who was recently admitted to the bar, and he stated there is now an emphasis on the win-win model in the training of law students.

WIN-LOSE VS. WIN-WIN

Two Biblical examples illustrate the difference between win-lose and win-win strategies. One side is calling down fire to destroy, while the other side desires fire to bring insight and understanding. In a win-lose example James and John aim at an ultimate loss for the opposition:

> And when his disciples James and John saw it, they said, 'Lord, do you want us to tell fire to come down from heaven and consume them? (Luke 9:54)

Contrast the reaction of James and John to God the Father's reaction on the day of Pentecost. Here is the win-win example where confusion is replaced with understanding, hearing people speak in languages other than their own. This was an incredible sign of divine presence that produced a new level of understanding:

> When the day of Pentecost arrived, they were all together in one place. And suddenly there came from heaven a sound like a mighty rushing wind, and it filled the entire house where they were sitting. And divided tongues of fire appeared and rested on each one of them. And they were filled with the filled with the Holy Spirit and began to speak in other tongues as the Spirit gave them utterance. (Acts 2:1-4)

A SECOND BIBLICAL MEDIATION

In this Biblical example involving a conflict, the contrast highlighted is between the win-lose vs. win-win approach to mediation. The Bible expresses this distinction in the language of justice and mercy.

Sadly, in the first half of my life, when wronged, I would have the tendency to go to battle and to bring down fire to destroy my assumed enemy, as the story of David and Nabal illustrates. In 1 Samuel, we see an example of how we jump quickly from negotiation to calling down fire. David sent ten of his young men to Nabal to negotiate for provisions. There is a clear foreshadowing of how this will go down, in the description of Nabal and his wife Abigail. "The women was discerning and a beautiful, but the man was harsh and badly behaved; he was a Calebite." (1 Samuel 25:3c)

As predicted, Nabal dismisses David's men in a gruff manner. David's response upon hearing the news is to instruct his men to strap on swords to bring down the fire of intense pain on Nabal and company. However, the discerning action of Abigail saves them from the sword. She comes secretly to David to apologize for Nabal's conduct. Abigail offers repentance, David accepts and forgives, and even thanks her, for saving him from the bloodguilt of avenging himself.

Abigail's timely and discerning action to mediate surely is what St. Paul had in mind when he gave crystal-clear direction to the Corinthian church about the ill of Christians pursuing lawsuits against other Christians.

> I say this to your shame. Can it be that there is no one among you wise enough to settle a dispute between the brothers, but brother goes to law against brother, and that before unbelievers. (1 Corinthins 6:5,6)

I confess to "strapping on my sword" from time to time. When I was 28 and again when I was 47 I "lawyered-up." Having the lawyer write my antagonist a letter was a thinly disguised calling down of fire, outlining a scorched earth policy to shrivel up enemies and opponents. It is not surprising to me that in almost every mediation I am a part of someone is calling down fire to toast his or her enemy, a Cold War of having more threat power in your backyard pointed at your enemy's favorite cities. Consume your enemy, dismiss them, get them fired, excommunicate them, humiliate them, make them unemployable, shake the dust off, leave the church, or the bishop.

As I have hinted in the above list, calling down fire is not the sole prerogative of lawyers. I see bishops, clergy, and lay people firebombing their annoying and destructive lay people, clergy, and bishops. Conflict escalates when individuals fail to listen and do not understand their opponent's position. Instead they see them as enemies and then cut them off.

VISION FOR CONFLICT

So, who do we need present when all around is smoke and flames are rising? An Abigail would really help keep us men from shooting first and asking questions later. Abigail's discernment resulted in her being a visionary. She saw alternatives to a fiery outcome. She anticipated the work of the Holy Spirit coming down to enable people of different races to hear each other in their own tongue. It was Abigail's tongue, not her sword, that opened David's ear and then his heart.

A peacemaker is a Christian mediator who is a visionary. They see through a different lens than the average person. They see the high value that Scripture places on unity. They see how important unity is to Jesus as He pleads to the Father, "that they all may be may be one just as you, Father, are in me, and I in you, that they may be one even as we are one." (John 17:21,22)

A visionary has a deepened appreciation for the work of the Holy Spirit to convict all parties of their own contribution to broken relationships. They see with renewed eyes the power of confession and repentance as opposed to the carnage created by bringing down fire.

Mediators are conflict tolerant rather than conflict aversive. They see conflict differently. If you do a word association using the word conflict, what response do you get? Bad, dangerous, destructive, pointless, unproductive, hurtful, to be avoided, or leads to anger? My own observation after years of embracing conflict as a gift and opportunity are renewed relationships, the air is cleared, boundaries are maintained and healing occurs, the time spent is very productive. All are outcomes to be embraced.

Both visions of conflict come from experience and both are justified from past encounters, but both lead to very different places. The former leads to withdrawal, avoidance, concession, accommodation, and appeasing. Sadly, if one responds to life using the list of behaviors in the prior paragraph, one may create a self-fulfilling reality. But if one leans into conflict with the positive view of conflict you create a reality that is self-fulfilling, but radically different than the misery that comes from a negative vision of conflict.

Jesus appears to have a very positive view of conflict. One third of the Gospel writings record Jesus in conflict with the Pharisees and Sadducees. Jesus invites conflict, sets up conflict, and confronts his opponents. He uses conflict for teaching moments.

Jesus begins his ministry with a conflict in the wilderness with Satan and ends his life in conflict with King Herod, the Jewish High Priest, the Secular Roman emperor, and forces of darkness. Yet in the midst of embracing a call to face conflict Jesus says, "Peace I leave with you; my peace I give you." (John 14:27) Not only does Jesus remain at peace in the midst of conflict, he gets his ministry done and has enough peace to spare for everyone around himself.

A Christian mediator needs also to have such a grasp of their own vision of conflict that they sail into conflict with a non-anxious presence aboard. But the skilled mediator knows which conflicts to avoid and how to remain safe in the midst of intense conflict.

Wisdom and discernment are their rudder and compass.

LEVELS OF CONFLICT

It is vital to have a vision for conflict that enables one to rise above the depressing depths of a conflict. At the same time one needs to understand the depth or entrenchment to which a conflict may deteriorate.

Author Speed Leas defines five levels of conflict, all the way from focus on just getting a solution to spiraling out of control in the desire to bring fire down on your enemies.

Level I

A Problem to Solve

Objectives are clear with some anger, but the focus is on a solution.

Level II

Multiple Disagreements

a) Self-protection, not getting hurt.
   1. Guardedness vs. openness. Sarcastic overtones.
b) Specifics shift to generalizations. We have lost the facts.
c) Compromise is sought to diminish the conflict.

Level III

Contest

a) Win-lose outcome seems inevitable.
b) Truth is distorted.
c) Language of putting people in their proper place.

Level IV

Fight or Flight

a) Objective to hurt opponent and/or to get rid of them.
b) Language full of principles, truth, and justice.

Level V

Intractable Situation

a) Singular objective to get rid of your opponent.

Leas' insightful evolution of conflict management demonstrates the move to calling down fire to get rid of the opponent. He also names the middle phases of conflict as the contest stage of win-lose.

Mediation is of course designed to be a win-win option for both parties. In the chapters that follow the hope is to bring creative win-win solutions to the real issues we encounter in the life of faith within the church.

See Appendix One for a fuller exposition of Speed Leas' thinking.

Two

The Person of the Mediator

By Bishop Trevor Walters

Your past shapes the way you view conflict and provides a default way of responding to it. The good news is training and counseling can change this predisposition. But if one fails to recognize how one has been shaped by a dysfunctional experience one will continue to do the same thing expecting a different result (the definition of insanity).

Family History

If your parents kept order by rules, one is more prone to seek rules in one's world to provide order. So if someone breaks the rules one will deem it right to administer the right amount of punishment to restore order. One will likely resonate with the prosecuting attorney role. If your parents kept order by love, one will seek to find a loving solution in one's adult world. Mediation calls your name!

If your father was harsh and rules were unbending and your mother would plead on your behalf you will likely identify with the defense attorney. If rescuing calls your name during mediation watch out. Remember, confession is the last option of a defense attorney and the first option for a Christian. A Christian mediator's first call is to invite the participants to take responsibility for their own sinful behavior that contributed to the level of conflict evident.

My own discovery that my childhood had conditioned me for rescuing happened in 1981 at the age of 32. The Canadian Association of Pastoral and Professional Educators held an inter-personal training session in Calgary. I attended the session and during the training, my wheels fell off! Let me explain. To become a specialist in Pastoral Counseling meant running the gamut of Interpersonal Relationship training (IPR). IPR entailed 90 minutes of torture. It was a free-flowing, unstructured group session to expose one's inner conflicted workings. We all dreaded our Tuesday afternoon bloodletting session. I suspect we all had our inner conflicts. On this particular day a tough priest named Geoff was, in my opinion, going after a blind man in the group called John. John appeared to be suffering at the hands of Geoff, who I say again appeared to be confronting him over some issue that happened earlier in the week. I could not resist my calling to be a rescuer, a white knight riding into the fray. I stepped between them, not quite literally, but enough to get the unwanted attention of the therapist, née torturer.

Here is my rescue example.

What are you doing Trevor?

I was trying to help John, I muttered in a low voice.

Do you think John needed your help? shot back the therapist.

Well, Geoff seemed to be going after him?

Do you want to ask John if he needed your help?

Probably not, I said under my breath.

This was not going to end well, but I had no idea why I was so reluctant to ask John if he needed my help.

John, did you need my help? I asked in a timid, self-doubting voice.

Drum roll, lights turn on full and every eye is upon me, awaiting my demise, or so it felt.

NO, I DID NOT. In fact, I was wondering what on earth you were doing, pronounced John.

A dead silence filled the room along with a stunned Trevor. I had been *tasered* by John's retort. My body went into spasm, my breathing was labored, and my sight was foggy. All was a blur especially on the ride home as I gazed out upon a world where my past perceptions lay in tatters. For me, victims were victims and I was here to rescue them. But now in less than 90 minutes of IPR I wondered if victims were really victims as I had supposed them to be.

Oddly enough, I began to see myself as being a victim needing rescuing. My past role had been to take issue with the persecutors of the victims and to bring down righteous fire on them. What if conflict did not need to be avoided, because the *Geoffs* of this world could handle conflict, and it was too often the *Trevors* that could not? Clearly I needed to find a way to handle conflict without polarizing the players as victims, rescuers, and persecutors.

That day in 1981 birthed the foundation of my healthier career in mediation. It took another 25 years to catch the vision that conflict is not chaos! So I the question: What motivates you to be a peacemaker?

a) Is there a motivation in mediation to avoid conflict?

b) Are you driven by the need to bring rules to bear to restore order?

c) Does it fulfill a need to be a rescuer?

d) Does keeping everyone happy motivate you?

e) Do you have a desire for unity at all costs?

f) Can you walk away from the desire to mediate a conflict when it is a discipline issue and not a mediation issue?

g) In a conflict do you over identify with: 1) those in authority 2) those who have no power 3) neither?

If you are saying, "No, my motives are not at issue with my being a peacemaker," then let's take a look at the preferred qualities of mediators.

TWELVE QUALITIES OF AN EFFECTIVE MEADIATOR

In this section we will take a look at twelve qualities of an effective mediator. Study them and see how you might utilize them with clients.

1. An Anointing to Mediate

A qualitative difference can be seen between a person who is anointed by God and one who is not. You cannot measure God's anointing, but one knows when it is present. From a human perspective one's passion for unity in the church maybe a characteristic of God's anointing. From a divine perspective one senses that God is present in the mediator.

The Holy Spirit provides power, a charisma that is operative in addition to the God given skill of the reconciler. The force therefore behind the initiative is not coercion, but cooperation with the Holy Spirit. Instead of a heavy hand the weight of the Holy Spirit presses in on the participants. Conviction comes from God rather than the mediator shaming participants into submission. There is no pitting one group against another as I have seen in so-called expert mediators. Instead, it is the power of God.

2. Discernment

Christian mediators have the advantage of accepting help from on high! In 1 Corinthians Paul describes nine spiritual gifts. (1 Corinthians 12:1-10) Paul discovered that the gifts of discernment and wisdom were given to him for the work of his ministry. Given that peacemaking is at the heart of ministry it stands to reason that God would give mediators an abundance of these gifts. Discernment does not flow out of a sharply focused mind; rather it flows directly from God to the minister who is open to being led by God. The recipient therefore has one ear to the conflict and another to God saying under their breath, "Lord what are you saying to us about this conflict?"

When I step into mediation, it is commonplace to be overwhelmed by how far this conflict has escalated. The participants want the other side removed (British understatement) and my task is to get them to forgive and make up. This appears to be the definition of impossible. I find myself saying to myself, "Why did I agree to do this to myself?" But I believe that God has provided an opportunity for me to participate in solving this disagreement.

I mouth the words, "Lord help, I am in trouble, give insight to bring the Light of Christ to end this darkness and hatred. Use me as an instrument of your peace."

Empathy alone at this point does not make mediation successful. Consequently, it is necessary to map out the dynamics of what is going on in conflict and how to shift the perspective from problem people to problem solving. Of course, one's learning road maps aid immensely, but it is a Holy Spirit moment that gives the big breakthrough.

My testimony is that God's gifts of knowledge and discernment have made all the difference in successful mediation outcomes. Scripture constantly presses me to seek, knock, and ask when in need. He always responds and His response is always a blessing.

3. Conflict Tolerant

Two polar opposite responses exist when it comes to how one reacts to conflict. You are conflict tolerant or the opposite, conflict aversive. If you are conflict aversive and shy away from conflict, you will burn out in the first month of being a mediator. Mediation would place one in such a place of inner turmoil that one would be at risk of prematurely rushing to a solution, to end the awful conflict.

I have learned a great deal about tolerating conflict from Dr. Scott Peck in his wise book, *To a Different Drum*. Peck explores how communities handle conflict. His research led him to identify four distinct conflict stages as groups wrestle with disagreements. They are:

a) Pseudo Community

b) Chaos

c) Emptying

d) True Community

In stage one (Pseudo Community) if a community is determined to avoid conflict, they will accentuate all that they have in common. They will be conflict aversive at all costs, as chaos must be avoided at all costs. To avert slipping into facing irreconcilable differences the mediator should focus on issues that both parities can agree upon. Individual differences are downplayed, while what one has in common is spoken about. This may result in one talking about the weather or the game last night on TV. So the community appears to have no conflict, but the price of being Pseudo Community is trivial and unsubstantial conversation.

Pseudo Community is very hard to maintain and the inevitable occurs. A dreaded difference breaks out of the shackles and the community is faced with how to deal with this frightening new information. The community is thrown into Chaos. They begin to ask all sorts of questions of one another. Examples are: How could you think so differently about who should be president? How could you like that sort of music in church? How could you feel that way about our mother? It is rather appalling that even in one's own home someone could believe something diametrically opposed to what I believe.

Whether one stays in Chaos or jumps back to Pseudo Community depends on whether one is conflict adverse or conflict tolerant. If it is the former, one will find a way of getting back to Pseudo Community ASAP. If one can tolerate the chaos believing it is necessary and healthy, one will find a very different path to real community, namely that of Emptying. Whereas a conflict-avoiding community responds to chaos by prematurely wanting to fix, solve, or heal the differences.

I had a perfect opportunity in a former parish to practice Scott Peck's theory of how staying in chaos can lead to real community. Two candidates were shortlisted for a position. The leadership team met to decide which candidate should be appointed. On the first vote we had a fifty-fifty split. We were divided over who should be called. We were a little surprised at how differently we each perceived the candidates. People spoke in animated ways about the obvious virtues of their candidate. Shock was registered in how one could possibly not see why their person was the right choice.

Sensing that chaos was looming for our community, I remembered Scott Peck's theory. Sure enough, to avoid the differences some now moved to impose a premature fix, solve, or heal. Some used pejorative language to describe the opposition's views. It was time to take a stand and to give my Scott Peck speech to try to provide a new perspective on selecting the best candidate.

I said, "Living in this division might be really important for our leadership team to see how well we can maintain unity whilst fundamentally disagreeing with some members here. Perhaps the health of our community at the end of this process is more about living with different views than finding the ideal candidate."

I succeeded in buying some time, but it was short-lived. I suggested that we go home and pray for a week and meet again for another vote. We came back together only to find that those voting for candidate A, now had switched to B, and those voting for B had switched to A.

The chaos of a fundamental difference remained, but we had turned a very significant corner. We had entered into stage 3, Emptying. Both sides, out of respect for the opinion of the other, had changed sides. To cut a long story short the process lasted two months. But at the end of the day we developed a new decision-making process: modified consensus. A candidate was appointed who turned out to be superb, and our leadership team never forgot the benefit of staying in the chaos, waiting for God's purpose to be revealed.

My natural tendency is to see chaos as a crisis. I have been unlearning that personal response from my past baggage, one of the poignant things I learned from my mediator training in Florida.

I had heard stunning reports of a certain mediator with a practice in a large city in Florida. Alas, he had a six-month waiting list to get an observation spot alongside him. I decided that his reputation was worth the wait.

The actual mediation that I sat in on was a common situation. One company wanted $120,000 for unpaid bills. The defendant believed that materials had not been delivered and that the actual amount due was $20,000. After an hour and a half of Henry Kissinger-style shuttle diplomacy, going between two rooms, we had sufficient movement so that all were optimistic that in the next 30 minutes we'd be on the way home with a mediated settlement.

Then the crisis hit—or at least I certainly knew it to be a crisis. The defendants suddenly announced that from $90,000 they were dropping back to $20,000 because they simply could not pay the second and third installments agreed upon in the last 90 minutes. Chaos threatening to consume us and to destroy the ground gained in mediation.

"Okay," said the esteemed mediator and he strode down the corridor to inform the other group.

This was too much for me, as I wondered why the mediator was so unfazed and calm. I ran after him, caught his sleeve and tugged vigorously before he disappeared into the inferno of the other group's explosive response.

"Isn't this a crisis?" I whispered. "Only if you want it to be," said the mediator quite indifferently. Then seeing my skepticism, he felt compassion toward me and explained his serenity. But I was shocked by what he said. "Look, I will be paid the same amount today, whether I settle this or not!" He walked off leaving me reeling. Was he so mercenary that he did not care about the outcome? I later concluded he knew that he was only as good as the people before him allowed him to be, given their lack of flexibility. "Wow," I exclaimed to myself. I don't function that way. I take all the responsibility for an outcome no matter who the players are or how they behave.

I left you hanging. How did the so-called crisis turn out to not be a crisis? Our master mediator entered the room and said: "You are not going to like this, but they have changed their offer and reverted back to their starting position!"

There was silence for just a second, until the other party acted just as I had predicted. It lasted far too long for my comfort level, but clearly not for the mediator's. Indeed his non-anxious presence was like a magnet. Finally, they were vacuumed up into his magnetic attraction. They turned on him and said, "So what is going on?"

"Well, you know that they are in receivership and that they agreed to pay $20,000 now and in successive months the difference. But the next company that they owe money to will meet them next week, and so any ability to pay beyond today is unreliable. In fact, the only real money is what you get today."

The leader admitted that yes. they were aware of the company being in receivership and agreed therefore with the mediator's assessment of what was real money. Further expletives that followed would ignite these pages if typed. Nevertheless they said as a last attempt to avoid the ensuing chaos, "Well, we don't have authority to settle for that low a figure."

"Would you like me to give you space so you can make a phone call?" A begrudging, fearful "yes" was returned, barely louder than a whisper. Ten minutes later we had a signed deal for the starting amount. And no one died or was murdered. So, I had to admit it was not a crisis. The mediator had stepped into the chaos unwilling prematurely to fix, solve, or heal it prematurely. Instead, he gave permission for them to be in chaos when he said, "You are not going to like this!"

4. Skilled Listener

One might be Conflict Tolerant because one listens to conflict with indifference. To be deeply present in the chaos puts the mediator in a different league.

The importance of this attribute is clear, given that a whole chapter is dedicated to this skill set. Effective listening builds confidence in those working with you. If the mediator does not seem to comprehend an issue, you have a strike one. Three failures to hear what is being said and you are out.

Letting the parties know that they have been heard builds not just confidence, but credibility. The mediator might well be able to help with the impasse if they actually know what it is. Rapport grows between mediator and client through the use of listening skills. This skill is foundational in all that is to follow in mediation.

5. Persona of Authority

When one has no power to mandate an agreement between the parties, one certainly needs to find power within to influence a settlement. In a hostile environment where people and parties are locked in fixed positions, it takes someone of significant influence to catalyze change. There are certain professions that rely upon influence to effect change. One may not have authority to make a person do something, but nonetheless the person will listen and consider carefully what is being said to them because they respect the knowledge and ability of the individual. Doctors cannot make a patient take a prescription, but it is highly likely the patient will do because of the position and persona that doctors have in society.

Within the church, certain positions similarly carry influence. The offices of Canon, Archdeacon, and Bishop within Anglicanism are respected. The denomination has provided credibility to the individuals with these offices that cause the adherents to take note. Even when a person holding one of these offices is outside of their jurisdiction and has no formal authority, they still have significant influence.

When conducting mediations in Christian circles, my church credential is as important as my civil credential. I am listened to because I am a bishop, even if my logic is weaker than someone who is not a bishop. At one level this is highly dangerous and plainly wrong; however, one needs all the help one can get when mediating in the lion's den.

In other denominations, District Superintendents bring the denomination's stamp of approval with them as they seek to mediate. However, in a denomination that is principally congregational vs. Episcopal, the level of influence from a District Superintendent can be less weighty.

People in conflict do not listen even at the best of times, so why should they listen to you, the mediator? The answer is that society expects them to listen to you. Doctors, lawyers, and university professors, for example, are leaders in society who command an audience. Within the Christian church, certain ranks carry more authority and command more attention.

In the Anglican Church, an Archdeacon is probably the lowest rank that would be effective in being listened to in a mediation context. However, if a priest or pastor were a lawyer or barrister in their professional life prior to being ordained, they are more likely to be perceived as having the right to mediate a conflict.

Personally, I have been surprised at how responsive people are to my being a bishop. The office of bishop gives authority to call people together. At the commencement of the mediation, I ask people to discern what sin they have added to the mix. That is an important question and must be attended to if the basis of Christian meditation is to be established.

Lawyers naturally bring an authority from being equipped and called to the bar. One ignores a lawyer at one's peril. When they offer an opinion about a legal matter, their opinion carries more weight than does a person with no legal training. Given that mediation is conducted in the backyard or, more accurately, the front entrance of the law courts, lawyers are an obvious choice to conduct Christian mediations.

6. Assertiveness

Having authority allows the mediator to interject in the midst of conflict and temporarily take control. You may have authority, but one needs to feel at ease in exercising it. One has to be free from people pleasing to be effective as a mediator. Critiquing the strength and weaknesses of either party's argument assists them to see when their demands are not realistic.

If the parties remain stuck in their fixed positions, it might be necessary to call an impasse. Calling a halt to the mediation requires courage and confidence on behalf of the mediator. My experience shouts that calling an impasse is not popular. As a result, participants may reframe your job description as a mediator to include responsibility for solving the conflict.

When control has been lost, the mediator must take over the runaway freight train. The moment the train is back within the speed limit, the mediator may vacate the driver's seat. Therein lie two perils. You may not get the train under control, and negative tone controls the meeting.

The argument, which says I am not a leader in control, goes out the window when one or more (often more) controlling people hijack the meeting. It is then that Hersey Blanchard's circumstantial leadership insight comes into play. It is not what sort of leader you are, but what kind of leader the present circumstance requires. A meeting with control freaks requires the mediator to be more controlling than the dominating person(s). The mediator must show strength and take the reins out of their hands.

Being a mediator is not for the faint of heart. I detest being loud and controlling, but I know that is what certain mediation situations call me to do redirect the discussion.

Years ago, I was mediating a conflict between two church groups that were at war. At the beginning of the meeting one of the participants, head of a large corporation, stated that his intent in the meeting was not to criticize but to understand what was going on. Thirty minutes into the meeting he had done nothing but criticize the other side and had turned the mediation into a court of interrogation.

Reluctantly, I interrupted him and reminded him of his stated intent at the beginning of the meeting, followed by the observation that he had proceeded to criticize something every time he had spoken. I concluded by asking which of those two approaches did he wish to continue.

Much to everyone's surprise and relief, he did not say another word for the rest of the meeting. We were then able to gain a much deeper understanding of the issues and come up with lasting solutions to move beyond the impasse.

He was equally in shock; perhaps as a corporate head he had never been spoken to quite that forcefully. For the rest of the meeting I had numerous self-doubts about my being highly assertive and perhaps slightly confrontational. Those doubts continued, despite the successful outcome, until a year later the corporate head happened to mention that he had cited the mediation as a model of how to deal with a difficult situation.

7. Non-Anxious Presence

Being assertive can at times flow out of being anxious; this is not a good plan. But assertive action and a state of being non-anxious is a winning combination. Strength combined with a peaceful spirit is compelling. After all, there is an over-abundance of angst in the room. Someone who is without fear is a gift. A non-anxious presence is a magnet that draws people in. They are eager to know what your views are concerning this conflict, given that one appears to be the most rational, objective person in the room.

The chance of effecting change for good is greatly enhanced when one's assertiveness flows out of a non-anxious presence. When one's non-anxious presence is observed, and how could you miss it in a raging sea, the participants want you at the helm. This peaceful presence begs a reason how come you could be so settled when most others are unsettled.

It goes back to having a vision for conflict. One's quiet spirit is not coming out of indifference, but out of a passion to see how this conflict be resolved. The immediacy of the conflict being resolved pales in comparison with how the Gospel will go forward in creating a healthy future with peace. My peace in the midst of conflict flows out of the knowledge that folks are distracted from the main thing, and it is my privilege to steer them back on course.

An authentic non-anxious presence rises up as a result of faith in God. But the effect is amplified by the Holy Spirit's presence in this conflict. So, I have one ear to the Holy Spirit and the other ear to the conflict. I am excited about how God will speak into this mess. I am expectant as to how God's power will be made perfect in the midst of our brokenness. If my non-anxious presence were a disposition I had to muster up within myself as a technique, I believe I might run the risk of appearing arrogant or disengaged.

If one has set up mediation as an opportunity to listen to God as well as to each other, one has introduced into this context the ultimate non-anxious presence, God himself. How many times did Jesus say, "be not anxious" or "why are you afraid because you do not have enough faith?"

The great promises in the farewell discourse of John's Gospel culminate in the promise that "peace I leave with you." The promise of peace provides great comfort when dealing with conflict.

When the mediator brings faith and peace into a conflict, their presence radiates the light of Christ and is perceived as a non-anxious presence. So, what happens when you have the level of peace that Jesus had in a storm?

He was able to sleep in the back of the boat while the disciples were bailing for all they were worth. (Luke 8:22-25) You get woken up by the disciples who know you know something they don't. They wake you up and plead with you to care about the storm they are in. The fact that Jesus is sleeping begs an explanation. His non-anxious presence is like a gravitational pull of a magnetic field in that draws one into the process.

Mediators should not leave home without having this disposition in their spirit, soul, and psyche. Before mediators leave home they should earnestly ask for the

Lord's presence and the Holy Spirit's guidance.[1] Recall the experience of Moses on Mount Horeb as his face began to glow as God was with him. One should enter the mediation with the presence of God reflecting from one's face. This provides a non-anxious presence and sometimes little do they know the Holy Spirit is at work.
The observed result is powerful and has a major impact..

8. Sense of Humor

Humor alongside a non-anxious presence is a great way to de-escalate excess emotion. Joking too much can backfire with disastrous results if the parties feel that the humor says that the mediator is not taking their concerns with the utmost seriousness. Hence, humor too early in the process is not advised. If the parties have decided that one genuinely cares about them and their needs, then some humor can be of enormous help to lighten the mood. Humor can find a helpful place when combined with paradoxical intention. By creating a scenario about the present situation that escalates the outcome to outrageous proportions, one hopes that people will laugh and see that one needs a better sense of proportion. Again, the risk reward of such a strategy must be weighed carefully. One may not recover from a failed paradoxical intention!

If the mediator has demonstrated a non-anxious presence with Biblical foundation, he or she can afford a little humor to lower the anxiety, fear, and tension swirling around the room. A humorous comment when the tension

---

[1] Judge George Peagler suggests that the Prayer of St. Francis could well be considered the Mediator's Prayer

is elevated can dissipate the angst. Better by far to mock oneself than another. It is likely game over if one does the latter. Not taking yourself too seriously is a subtle invitation for others to go and do thou likewise.

British dry wit is my favorite form of humor, so mediation is where I try to employ it. Dry wit and sarcasm, the lowest form of wit, are not the same thing. Sarcasm has a caustic and cutting edge that burns and wounds. Check that "humor" at the door.

I recall saying in a mediation session, having unearthed twenty-four reasons for why this conflict was a perfect storm, "Well, I don't think you missed any known reasons. This is a perfect storm and you have got the waterfront covered!" This was a lighthearted way of conveying the inevitability of a conflict in a way that was not depressing, but informative. In effect it deflects away from the belief that a person on either side is the reason for the problem.

People in conflict loose their sense of humor and forget to fun. The mediator can help bring life back from gloom as a kindness to the people involved. Mediators should bring life more abundant, and season peace with joy.

Naming the complexity of the problem will nuance the perspective from a black and white picture.

9. Ability to Represent Those in Authority and Those Who are Powerless

One must win the confidence of the person in authority and also with those lower in the hierarchy, without getting triangulated. It is so easy to fall into the Kaufman's Drama Triangle of rescuer, victim, and persecutor. If the conflict is between a bishop and a priest, the default triangulation is the bishop as the persecutor and the priest as victim. But if one has the position of needing to maintain good order, one might reverse the triangulation and see the bishop and his authority as under attack and therefore the victim.

How do you protect the hierarchy and allow individuals with less authority a sense that they've been heard?

It is assumed by the lower-power person that as mediator, one represents the bishop, as in most cases it is the bishop who has engaged a mediator. My own approach is to explain this dynamic to the bishop and ask if he would like to hear the story as soon as possible from the lower-power person. Several contacts with the lower-power person, and dropping into the conversation, "Well I don't know about that. I have not talked to the bishop about that yet," helps to reassure them that you the mediator do not solely represent the bishop.

However, in so doing, one cannot level the hierarchy so that the mediation is between equal parties. There is a level of complexity here that does not usually exist in the same way in civil mediation unless one is mediating in the same company. There is an acute tension in managing these two realities and needs. Both opinions count, but the hierarchy must be honored and respected.

10. Capable of Articulating a Plan

Empathy, humor, and a non-anxious presence only go so far. The end game is providing a plan to move forward by solving problem(s) and thereby maintaining healthy relationships. One's capacity to think outside the box creatively imagining possible solutions is invaluable. There is, however, still a box much larger than the one in civil mediation. The authority of the Bible and the forgiveness of Christian morality may limit freethinking when problem solving.

Those who enjoy problem-solving excel in mediation. I have however already cautioned that this activity must not be a means to avoid dealing with Peck's stage of Emptying. Premature solving prevents adequate exploration of the nature of the problem.

The course I taught at Athabasca University is Problem Solving in Groups. The course emphasizes that most of the time spent resolving conflict resolution should be spent in problem definition vs. problem solving. Consider that many conflicts cease to be a problem when the reason(s) behind them are adequately discovered. So often in industry you find that speedy solutions require another solution in a few months' time. Problems carefully researched at the early stage of discovery often result in long-term solutions.

An apocryphal story told in almost every mediation course illustrates that an inadequate understanding of a problem leads to an inferior solution.

Two individuals are following two different recipes in the same kitchen. At a critical moment in the preparation both people conclude that they need an orange. Both arrive at the refrigerator at the same time to discover that there is only one orange. Both assert their need for said orange. Tension rises and in an attempt to save a fight they cut the orange in half and go back to their cooking.

Ultimately, they discover that they have differing needs concerning the orange. One recipe needs the rind while the other needs the juice.

The illustration demonstrates that a compromise may not be the ideal solution. The cooks failed to explore or define the problem, so their actual needs for the orange were not revealed. When they discovered they had complementary needs rather than competing needs for the orange they realized that a different resolution could have easily resolved the conflict.

If the mediator fails to offer a plan one party may attempt to resolve the issue by forcing a solution on the other party. At this point the mediator needs to encourage them to ask for more information

11. Multiple Strategies for Resolving Conflict

One solution does not fit all. In Chapter 6, various approaches to mediation will be explored. Every situation is different, and every person that is conflicted is unique. Attempting to process people through a system, versus being guided by the best and most creative process is limiting. A competent mediator will have a number of tools to assist them in resolving conflict.

12. Willingness to Fail

Calling an impasse is not necessarily a failure. It can be the stimulus to rethink the problem. However, if the mediator takes on the responsibility of getting the conflict resolved, then there is a high degree of potential failure lurking. A mediator once told me that the mediator is only as good as the clients they work with. If the mediator has an uncooperative party, there is little one can do to get movement toward a resolution. An impasse is almost inevitable.

I allude again to the mediator who said to me, "I am going to get paid the same whether I get this resolved or not!" I have to confess that in a difficult mediation, I have offered this statement more than once under my breath, hoping that I would not be heard. It is not about being mercenary but about not taking responsibility for the outcome. This whisper to myself helps me deal with the sense of failure of not successfully mediating the problem.

I was once mediating a conflict between two parishes sharing a priest. Both wanted the Sunday service time at 10:00 am. After two hours, I declared an impasse, as I saw little movement in one of the parties. I suggested we meet again in two weeks. The Sunday following the Thursday meeting, I had a phone call at 2:00 pm. One of the parties called to tell me that the conflict had been resolved. I was shocked and even a little disappointed, that they did not need me to fix the problem. They explained how they had discussed the previous failure to resolve the problem with their parish that morning, after church. Their congregation had decided to give complete freedom to their leadership team to resolve the issue in any way that would help the other church. Hence, they had called the other church and signed off on a new time agreement for the services. My gut feeling in hearing the solution was that it would not last. I had no intention of interfering at this point because they had taken responsibility to resolve the problem, which for the time being was more important than the quality of the solution.

Sure enough, the solution held only for six months! We returned to mediation this time with both parties willing to flex. A new, more tenable solution was reached quickly, and it proved to be a permanent solution. A willingness on my part, to name our failure by calling an impasse led to a solution reached by them Chapter 3.

Three

Becoming an Artful Listener

By Jack Lewis

It can be stated, with practically no qualification, that people in general do not know how to listen. They have ears that hear very well, but seldom have they acquired the necessary aural skills that would allow those ears to be used effectively for what is called *listening*. These are the words of Dr. Ralph Nichols, known as the "Father of the Field of Listening," and Leonard Stevens, a writer and consultant, in an article titled "Listening to People" published in 1957.[2] Almost 60 years later, it seems Nichols's and Steven's comments (or laments) have never been truer.

"Now Hear This! Most People Stink at Listening" reads the title of a Scientific American article, an extract from *The Plateau Effect* (2013) by Bob Sullivan and Hugh Thompson who, among other things, infer "the average American has little time or energy to listen well as a result of being overworked, tethered to our work iPhones and

---

[2] Ralph Nichols and Leonard Stevens, "*Listening to People*," *Harvard Business Review* (September 1957).

Blackberries, and often having no or an unhealthy work life balance."[3]

I think it is safe to say the U.S. 2016 presidential campaign and election highlighted how poorly many of us listen, which in turn has contributed to the pervasive political divisiveness we are experiencing.

"*What we've got here is failure to communicate.*"[4]

Eric Liu, a former speechwriter and deputy domestic-policy adviser for President Bill Clinton, suggests a path forward for the healing that we seem to desperately need. Not surprisingly, the first step on that proposed path is listening. And when Liu says *listening* he doesn't mean a "debater's listening" in which the listener pays just enough attention to prepare her rebuttal. Rather, he means "radically compassionate listening: without judgment, without response."[5]

Along the same lines, in a recent article "Listening to America" in California Chico State University's student newspaper, Evan Roberts and Dongyoung Won issue a call for "purposeful listening" to help heal the "hatred and divide present in America's current political climate."[6]

---

[3]*Scientific American*, May 3, 2013.

[4]Strother Martin's (Captain, Florida Road Prison #36) admonition to Prisoner Luke (Paul Newman) in the1967 movie Cool Hand Luke.

[5]Eric Liu, "Americans Don't Need Reconciliation-They Need To Get Better At Arguing" *The Atlantic* (November 1, 2016)

[6]Evan Roberts and Dongyoung Won, "*Listening to America*," *The Orion* (December 8, 2016)

Sadly, poor listening is not limited to political circles. If you beg to differ, take some time this week to take careful note of as many conversations as you can and grade all the listeners in those conversations. Are the listeners resisting distractions, looking the speaker in the eye, concentrating on everything that is being said, asking insightful questions to help ensure their understanding of the speaker's message and feelings, and letting the speaker finish speaking?

THE ART OF LISTENING

According to Dr. Michael Nichols, author of *The Lost Art of Listening*, how we lost the art of listening is a matter of debate. However, Nichols believes it is incontrovertible that the loss of this art leaves us with "an ever-widening hole in our lives."[7]

Radically compassionate listening. Purposeful listening. These notions sound daunting, don't they? And they seem even more daunting when you consider the average person suffers from the delusion that he or she is a good listener.[8]

Upon reading Adam McHugh's, *The Listening Life: Embracing Attentiveness in a World of Distraction* recently, I recognized that I have far to go to become a competent listener, never mind a radically compassionate listener or an artful listener. "Listening," so McHugh writes, "is foundational to what it means to be human." As a result, it

---

[7] Michael P. Nichols, *The Lost Art of Listening: How Learning to Listen Can Improve Relationships* 2nd ed. (New York: The Guilford Press, 2009), p159

[8] Steven Sample, *The Contrarian's Guide to Leadership* (San Francisco: Jossey-Bass, 2002.)

has become clear that much has been said to me that I have not completely understood or even heard at all.

This is a sobering realization and one that I have committed to work on. It also was sobering to read about and reflect upon God's prominence in our listening lives. I already knew intellectually that we have a listening God who has given us the gift of listening. However, what hadn't sunk in is that we are called to use our gift of listening in the service of serve others.[9]

McHugh got my attention when he pointed out in his book's Introduction that "throughout the Bible listening is the central act of the people of God", "the centerpiece of Israel's prayer life, the *Shema* begins with the word hear," and "listening is the first act of discipleship as fisherman drop their nets and follow when Jesus calls."[10]

If this is starting to resonate with you, there is something else I need to tell you. It seems listening well is hard work and requires practice, apparently lots of practice.[11] William Ury, in his exceptional TEDx Talk, "The Power of Listening,"[12] submits that genuine listening needs to be learned and practiced every day. And to illustrate the level of work artful listening requires, the observations of Rob

---

[9] McHugh explores all facets of a healthy "Listening Life" and, in addition to encouraging his readers to listen to God and others he speaks to the importance of listening to scripture, creation, and our own lives.

[10] McHugh, *The Listening Life*, 10.

[11] Nichols, *The Lost Art of Listening*, 159.

[12] William Ury, "The Power of Listening," (TEDx, San Diego, 2015). TED (Technology, Entertainment, Design) is a media organization that posts talks online for free distribution, under the slogan "ideas worth spreading".

LaZebnik, television producer and writer for *The Simpsons* TV program, hit home for me when he said, "It's more fun to talk than to listen. Talking is like drinking a great Cabernet. Listening is like doing squats."[13]

THE UNARTFUL LISTENER

If you are someone who finds it useful to have the negative pointed out and explained, I have just the thing for you. It is Dr. Marie Hartwell-Walker's succinct and no-holds barred article, "*The Eight Habits of Lousy Listeners.*" These habits, which are sure to louse up a conversation in a hurry, produce various types of un-artful listeners.

- The distracted listener who tends to other things when you are speaking, such as checking out his latest text or thinking about what to have for lunch.
- The listener who is planning his response while you are speaking, and who is prone to speak before you finish speaking.
- The ball stealer who, upon hearing you went to the Grand Canyon, can't wait to tell you about his trip to the Grand Canyon or one-ups you and tells you about his Paris vacation.
- The subject changer who steers the conversation in a different direction before you are ready to do so. The impatient listener who hurries you along and who may look at his watch or say, "Uh-huh, uh-huh, uh-huh," a lot.

---

[13] Rob Lazebnik, "*It's True: You Talk Too Much*," The Wall Street Journal (October 4, 2013).

- The listener who has lousy nonverbal skills and who provides little or no meaningful eye contact and/or affirmation.
- The easily offended listener, who will tend to see criticism or blame in the most innocent of discussions."
- Listeners who "are quick to offer advice, even when it hasn't been asked for."[14]

Not surprisingly, the traits of these lousy listeners spring from a focus on self and not a focus on the listener. They may as well be telling you, "No, no, I'm listening. It just takes me a while to process so much stupid all at once."[15]

LISTENING ARTFULLY

In his book *The Contrarian's Guide to Leadership*, Steven Sample says, "Listen first, talk later; and when you listen, do so artfully."[16] Simple, straightforward, but not so easy without some guidance. Dr. Michael Nichols provides these helpful "Guidelines for Good Listening" in his highly acclaimed *The Lost Art of Listening.*[17]

---

[14] Marie Hartwell-Walker, "*The Eight Habits of Lousy Listening,*" PsychCentral.com (2016).

[15] Sheldon Lee Cooper, PhD, ScD, a fictional character in the CBS television series *The Big Bang Theory*.

[16] Steven B. Sample *The Contrarian's Guide to Leadership*, (Jossey-Bass, 2002), 189.

[17] Nichols, *The Lost Art of Listening*, 152-153

1. Concentrate on the person speaking.
    - Set aside distractions.
    - Suspend your agenda.
    - Interrupt as little as possible. If you do interrupt, it should be to encourage the speaker to say more.
2. Try to grasp what the speaker is trying to express.
    - Don't react to just the words, listen for the underlying ideas and feelings.
    - Try to put yourself in the other person's shoes.
    - Try to understand what the other person is getting at.
3. Let the speaker know that you understand.
    - Use silence, reassuring comment, paraphrasing.
    - Offer empathetic comments.
    - Make opening-up statements (Tell me more, what else) versus closing-off statements (I get it; the same thing happened to me).

There are other well-written and helpful guidelines on developing good listening skills (e.g. *What Great Listeners Actually Do*[18]), most of which relate to important mechanical listening skills. Ah, but watch out! A problem arises "when listening is reduced to a laundry list of how-tos, as some

[18] Jack Zenger and Joseph Folkman, "*What Great Listeners Actually Do*," Harvard Business Review (July 14, 2016)

people make more of an effort to show that they're listening than to actually listen."[19]

Adam McHugh would take the "'list' out of listening."[20] "You can give a person all the tools for listening, you can teach him all the right techniques, you can introduce him to the fancy words, such as active listening, mirroring, paraphrasing, and repeating open-ended questions, but a person's listening ability is not determined by the techniques in his arsenal."[21]

McHugh is on a quest for a "listening heart"[22] which is what I suggest will help transform a good listener into an artful listener. What is a "listening heart"? It is a servant's heart and the opposite of a selfish heart. "The listening heart is one that seeks to give, to learn, to welcome, to serve... the listening heart seeks to be present, to be focused on something other than itself and to give its attention away."[23] And, according to Hugh MacKay, when we truly listen to someone we are being "remarkably generous" as we are giving them the gifts of understanding, acceptance, and taking them seriously.[24]

---

[19] Nichols, *The Lost Art of Listening*, 90.

[20] McHugh, *The Listening Life*, 135.

[21] Ibid, 135.

[22] Ibid, 136. Here McHugh references a portion of King Solomon's prayer for wisdom. "Give your servant therefore an understanding mind to govern your people, that I may discern between good and evil." (1 Kings 3:9 ESV). McHugh notes that in this passage "understanding mind" is the usual translation, but in the Hebrew, it is literally "a listening heart."

[23] Ibid, p137-138.

[24] Hugh Mackay, *Why Don't People Listen? Solving the Communication Problem* (Sydney: Pan Australia, 1994), p146.

Developing a listening heart sounds challenging and time-intensive. But Dietrich Bonhoeffer viewed it as ministry.

> "We do God's work for our brothers and sisters when we learn to listen to them. So often Christians, especially preachers, think that their only service is always to have to 'offer' something when they are together with other people. They forget that listening can be a greater service than speaking. Many people seek a sympathetic ear and do not find it among Christians, because these Christians are talking even when they should be listening." [25]

As I strive to become a better listener, even an artful listener, I plan to take these cues from Adam McHugh and Michael Nichols.

- Aim to listen to, not listen for. In your mannerisms and speech, extend an invitation to other people to settle in, be themselves and speak freely.[26]
- Remember the "scandalous premise that this conversation is not about you."[27]
- "An open question is gracious and curious, without a hint of control or agenda."[28]
- "Empathy is permission giving. Receptive, non-defensive listeners help get our feelings out."[29]

---

[25] Dietrich Bonhoeffer, *Life Together* (London: SCM, 1972), 75.
[26] McHugh, *The Listening Life*, 139.
[27] Ibid, 143.
[28] Ibid, 144.

- What defeats us isn't the provocative speaker but our own defensive response. The best way to master emotional reactivity is by having the courage to engage emotionally intense situations and tolerate the anxiety associated with that engagement."[30]
- The person who starts a sentence should be the one who finishes it."[31]
- Listening for understanding is slow. A good listener believes in taking the long route."[32]
- Listen for nonverbal clues, i.e. body language (gestures, eye contact, posture) and voice (tone, volume, speed, intensity).[33]
- Listen for "…authentic moments, those truly human moments when someone reveals herself to us, when the mask, even for a second, comes off and we meet the real person."[34]

A FINAL THOUGHT

We live in a culture that seems to desperately need more artful listeners. The road to becoming such a listener appears quite challenging. However, while listening well requires time, energy, patience and authenticity, it does not

---

[29] Nichols, *The Lost Art of Listening*, 177.
[30] Ibid, 179.
[31] Ibid, 159.
[32] McHugh, *The Listening Life*, 150.
[33] Ibid, 151.
[34] Ibid, 157-158.

seem to be complex at all. In his epilogue to *The Listening Life*, Adam McHugh reminds us all that there is no glory in listening. Yet, he also reminds us that it is a gift from a listening God, one that helps us grow into servants and disciples, and it is a precious and important gift we can offer others.[35]

[35] Ibid, 213-214.

Four

Active Listening Skills

By Bishop Trevor Walters

Let's take a step back to try to understand the science of communicating. What actually happens when someone speaks? The communicator is creating a unique code that is distinct from any other person. When one is actively listening, one is deciphering that code. To test their understanding the respondent may offer back the decoded message in their own words. One is thereby seeking to gain confirmation that they have accurately interpreted the code. If the two parts of communications are coding and decoding, then skilled listening focuses on decoding the message.

The unskilled listener may endure the humiliation of risking an interpretation only to have the coder denounce the attempt. So the un-artful respondent may stop risking, and end up, well, making useless grunts at inappropriate moments.

In this chapter I am going to focus on two forms of decoding in communication: *Paraphrasing* and *Reflective Listening*. When a successful clarification happens, the speaker will pause, make eye contact and communicate in effect: "That's right, you do get it!"

PARAPHRASING

Paraphrasing is one of the chief clarifying skills employed by successful mediators. By offering back to the parties a summary, in one's own words, the process is slowed sufficiently. This slowing allows for participants to reflect before piling on another argument. In addition, paraphrasing helps clarify for oneself and for others whether one understands what has been communicated.

When one fails to accurately paraphrase, the recipient will lose momentum, feel frustrated, and say something like: "No, that's not it at all!" Momentum is immediately lost, the mediator has then to make a second attempt to recapture the essence of the communication. (To get the idea of momentum in mediation picture a giant snowball being pushed along a snowy field. The moment it stops, the effort required to restart it is enormous, but once it's moving again, minimum effort is needed to keep the mediation moving along.)

Ah, but when a successful clarification happens the recipient will pause, make eye contact and acknowledge that you "get it." Thus the successful paraphrase builds up kinetic energy and propels the mediation process of communication in a positive direction.

The second use of paraphrasing is when there is an uncomfortable silence. Then it might be appropriate to say, "Lets recap what has been said. I think your three main points are...". This often provides an opportunity to restart the communication between parties. Here one is decoding more than sentences, but also the principles and purposes for which the individual codes serve merely as individual notes on a manuscript page. To be true to the metaphor, I could have said that paraphrasing is testing whether one has understood the themes and variations of what has gone on.

Paraphrasing is especially important when the mediation has physically separated the parties, and the mediator is carrying messages between the parties. I have witnessed mediators actually writing down what they have heard from one group before presenting an offer to the next group. Before leaving the one they may say: "This is what I am going to present to the other party. Is this what you want me to communicate?" Paraphrasing is a relatively simple skill, yet nevertheless a highly effective one and a very important "tool" for mediators.

The third use of paraphrasing is to help the coder reflect upon the current direction, so they can redirect the conversation if it is not serving the purpose. Paraphrasing provides the moment for a mid-course correction.

REFLECTIVE LISTENING

The greatest tool in the listener's toolbox is the skill of *Reflective Listening*. It is a skill utilized throughout the communication process, but requires a much higher degree of precision: A reflective response must accurately get the subject or content right, and identify the emotion attached to the event described. It limits the possibility that a message will be lost in translation.

Here are four levels of reflective listening, from not good at all (Level 1) to very good indeed (Level 4):

Level 1

The respondent provides an inaccurate description of the content of the communication, which is hurtful because it misidentifies the emotion in a way that could be demeaning.

Level 2

The respondent accurately identifies the content or subject matter but only partially identifies a surface emotion.

Level 3

The respondent captures the content and correctly identifies the emotion. (One doesn't have to name the content if it is implicitly understood.)

Level 4

The response accurately describes the content and the feelings. In addition, it opens a door for the coder to identify an emotion that was implied but not named in their response.

Returning to the snowball metaphor, it requires at least a Level 2.5 response to keep the mediation snowball advancing. A response that is less accurate than this will create an awkward moment with loss of momentum. The theory holds that one should be aiming for a Level 3 response. The problem with aiming for Level 4 (trying to provide an additive emotional factor) is that if one fails in this the response will plummet to a Level 2 at best. This may even be perceived as hurtful and result in a low Level 1 response.

When I was attempting to learn these skills in graduate school, among other aspiring counselors and psychologists, I was shocked by how difficult it was to reflect in a way that keeps the listening process moving. So often we lapsed into the old stale phrase, "What I hear you saying is...". Then there was a collective groan around the classroom as we realized how stereotypical that sounds.

Even worse was an empathetic grunt or sigh, "Ahhh yes," followed by "I understand." One dare not say, "I understand" if one hasn't really grasped the issue.

Case in point; A few days ago, I was having a very difficult time on the telephone with an airline agent over getting a particular seat. The small print indicated that I was eligible for it.

After many attempts to communicate my point to the agent, without her seeming to grasp the issue, she made the mistake of following the manual for appeasing a difficult frustrated customer.

She said in a sweet voice:

> "*Sir, I do understand your frustration.*"

To which I said,

> "*I am so grateful that you understand, but could you then explain to me why I am frustrated?*"

A pregnant pause was followed by a rather timid:

> "*Well, no sir, I can't*"

My response was,

> *"It does not help me when you say that you understand when you don't understand."*

It was time to take my frustration elsewhere.

How does a person express understanding without sounding like an *automated* counselor, i.e., "What I hear you saying is…".

The answer is by *inflecting* the last two or three words of the speaker's statement. This turns their statement into a reflective response. When successful, it raises the rating of the response to the desired Level 2.5 or higher.

To inflect is to raise one's voice significantly higher. If you are a musician that means moving up at least three notes higher. Inflecting turns a statement back on itself, posing a question that the coder is invited to confirm or deny. It represents the work of active listening.

I as the listener am working with you, keeping pace and neither lagging nor getting out in front of you.[36] It reassures the coder that I am tracking with them. Tracking inspires confidence to keep communicating.

REFECTIVE LISTENING SAMPLES

Sample A

The priest or pastor has just shared with the congregation that church giving for the year is $10,000 below budget. The bad news is that the diocese is

[36] The exception is if one has a rare prophetic word or word of knowledge that propels the momentum forward.

publishing the names of parishes that are behind on their contributions to the diocese.

Level 1 Response:

What's wrong with your fund-raising program?

Level 2 Response:

You have no money to pay the diocese!

Level 3 Response:

You're feeling powerless to pay what you don't have. (Last three words *inflected*)

Level 4 Response:

It feels like the bishop has no empathy for what it is like to be here in a parish. (last three words *inflected*)

Sample B

A church leader has raised the question of whether the parish would be better served by another pastor. They point out the age of the pastor as being close to retirement, and that the congregation itself is graying rapidly. They tell you the pastor doesn't like email much less Facebook as a means of communication.

Level 1 Response:

The pastor must be made to do email.

Level 2 Response:

An aging congregation does need a younger pastor.

Level 3 Response:

> You are anxious your current pastor is out of touch with his congregation.

Level 4 Response:

> You're wondering if a younger pastor would be more accessible.

Sample C

Two parishes share one pastor and both want their Sunday service to be at 10:00 a.m. Parish A does cannot get access to their rented building until 9:30 a.m. and has to be out by 11:30 a.m. Parish B is an older congregation that doesn't think they'll survive if services were before 10:00 a.m. Parish A says, "We've looked all over town for another space, and this is by far the best. If we can't have the 10:00 a.m. worship time we think the leadership will be overwhelmed!"

Level 1 Response:

> Both parishes will have to compromise!

Level 2 Response:

> You do not see any other options.

Level 3 Response:

> It looks like a hopeless situation if you can't get the 10:00 a.m. worship time.

Level 4 Response:

> Not getting the 10:00 slot could be the last straw.

Sample D (Practice)

A bishop is beside himself with the hostility of a parish to his leadership. He states, "I am ready to 'excommunicate' the parish and to cut them free from the diocese."

Level 1

Level 2

Level 3

Level 4

Sample E (Practice)

The rector of a church believes another bishop will better serve him and his "missional" parish. He states, "I need a bishop who 'gets it' about our church planting DNA. I think Bishop X would help us get us past our current plateau!"

Level 1

Level 2

Level 3

Level 4

Five

Benefits and Limits of Mediation

By Hon. George M. Peagler, Jr.

Mediation is not designed to replace discipline. Some years ago, one bishop was having a boundary conflict with another bishop, so he contacted Bishop Walters. He asked if Bishop Walters would be willing to mediate a conflict between himself and that bishop. Exploring the nature of the problem revealed that the other bishop had not followed accepted protocol. Bishop Walters suggested the way forward was not to mediate a discipline issue. It would be far better to invite a superior who could issue, in a professional manner, a cease and desist order to the offending bishop.

Limits of Mediation

Similarly, mediators should not seek to mediate principles. The application of a particular principle can be negotiated but not the principle itself, especially when it is Biblically based.

Example A

A conflict arises in a local church about the use of prophetic words in the church service. Mediation should not even attempt to address the validity of prophetic words. That is for the local priest and bishop to determine.

What does the use of prophetic words represent? To one group it could mean we are a bona fide charismatic church, whereas to another group it might mean we are not really Anglican. The mediator can most usefully engage the parties in a discussion of the underlying principles surrounding the presenting issue of using prophetic words, and the impact and application of prophetic words. Exploring how the use of prophetic words impacts each of the two groups could be quite valuable.

The mediator can explore what else could be seen in the existing service format that says that we are Anglican or charismatic or both. It may be the groups have shared interests in other aspects of the service that they value and that say we are both Anglican and charismatic.

What else could we do in the service to proclaim we are Anglican and charismatic, things that would be acceptable to both sides? Thinking outside the box with both parties can be fruitful in resolving an impasse of fixed positions.

Example B

A parish decides it wants to be under the authority of a different bishop. Disappointed expectation often leads to resentment, which in turn often leads to conflict. It may be that another bishop might be a better fit for the parish, whether in terms of churchmanship, church planting, personality, availability, or mission orientation. Yet the mediator must not enter the discussion of who would be the better bishop for the parish. By being neutral the mediator can help the parish, and their existing bishop, to better understand what each expects of the other.

Exploring the benefits to a p arish, diocese, or even a province of good oversight can change perspectives from what's best for the local parties to what's best for the denomination itself. False dichotomies, such as 'I must be under another bishop,' can be nuanced toward exploring what is it that is wanted from another that the existing bishop isn't providing. Indeed, it may be possible without changing horses to get support from the existing bishop along the lines of what the other might have to offer.

Example C

A parish is imploding in a division over whether the parish facility should be used for day care during the week. Half the members believe this is essential; the others believe it would curtail existing ministries and are therefore in totally opposed.

The mediator cannot be drawn into evaluating whether a day care center is a Biblical expression of social justice. That is a debate about principle, one that needs to be resolved between the pastor and bishop. The mediator can, however, explore with each group what a day care program would represent as a sign of their theology of social justice. What in the parties' histories forms their beliefs about it? Has it been assumed that history will repeat itself? In what other ways might the parish proclaim the underlying principles held by the opposing groups?

BENEFITS OF MEDIATION

The justice system in our country has benefited greatly from mediation. It provides an alternative to the court system for conflict resolution, while giving the participants the maximum possible influence for the outcome. It does so in a timely manner. Moreover, it increases the likelihood that the participants will gain a deeper understanding of their problem. The alternative of a getting a judge to understand the problem sufficiently to make a proper ruling is second best. Ending the conflict is only the short-term goal. The long-term goal is to get the causes of problems understood, so that in the future good problem-solving strategies can be applied in resolving disputes.

The biggest benefit of mediation over what the justice system offers lies in tutoring the parties in approaches to problem solving, wherein relationships are strengthened, healed and allowed to flourish. And mediation can save a fortune in time and money, especially when trained mediators volunteer their time and expertise to support the Christian community.

Indeed, more needs to be said about mediation resolving conflict in a timely manner. When a conflict goes to court the wait is perhaps six months to a year or more before the matter can get before a judge. If there are appeals it may be years before it is all over and done with. And perhaps the worst of it is that during all this time the people are in turmoil, stressed and spending money.

Bishop Walters (and his is one of many such stories) speaks from bitter experience about the loss of church buildings. The trial judge's decision had been contrary and launched four-years of appeals, a process that ended with an unfavorable decision of the Supreme Court. Protracted delays meant that people's anger and resentment at the justice system was kept at slow boil and created scars yet to fully heal.

I well remember a conversation in a courthouse elevator with one of the parties to a civil mediation. It was a few weeks before Christmas. The woman said, "I didn't get as much as I hoped, but it is worth so much to be able to let go of this thing and not take it into the Christmas season!"

Clearly the short-term goal was reached in that civil mediation. The decision did put the immediate issue to rest and it helped clear a path for Christmas. But unless long-term goals, in terms of mending patterns of thinking and emotions, were addressed and agreed (which I think was unlikely) the parties to that mediation remain vulnerable to more dust-ups down the road.

Six

Engaging With the Parties

By The Rev. Canon Jonathan Millard

Very often the situation between disagreeing parties has already reached something of an impasse by the time mediation is being contemplated. If they weren't stuck, they likely wouldn't need a mediator. Of course it's not always the case. Sometimes parties are savvy enough to realize that involving a neutral third party early on could be very helpful. For example, a divorcing couple that wants to avoid going to court if possible to save costs may engage the services of a mediator to resolve their case. This could be accomplished either formally or informally.

A. Getting to Mediation

Tragically, mediation is seldom the normal route disagreeing parties take to address their conflicts. This may be especially true in church disputes, particularly if clergy are involved. After all we who are clergy consider ourselves to be mediators. We know all about mediation, we think. Indeed, isn't mediation at the heart of the Gospel message? Christ is our mediator. We in the church are in the business of reconciliation, forgiveness, and healing. For a member of the clergy to admit they need a mediator is tantamount to admitting failure as a pastor.

It's one thing to be a dispassionate honest broker for people who come into the pastor's office with a problem. It is quite another if the pastor is part of that problem.

Sadly, what so often happens is that pastors try to fix whatever it is that needs fixing and they fail. Then the dispute escalates. The stakes are raised, and by the time mediation is on the table it's a last-ditch attempt to resolve matters before permanent and damaging consequences ensue. In civil matters mediation is often the last attempt to resolve a dispute before all-out war in the courts. Mediation of a church dispute may be the last effort at settlement before someone leaves the church, a leader resigns, or a leader is formally disciplined and/or removed from his or her position.

All this is to say that mediators need to be aware that by the time they have been asked to serve they will likely going into a veritable hornet's nest, facing a situation fraught with failed attempts at resolution, all exacerbated by boatloads of fear of the possible outcome of mediation. This can lead to low or false expectations of what mediation is all about. And the parties will tend to focus all their frustration, fear, and failure onto you the mediator. You the might even be perceived as a hatchet man.

All this is to underscore the importance of a mediator knowing what they are getting themselves into prior to the first contact or entering into a contract.

Understanding the Subtext

But more than needing to be forewarned, the mediator needs to be *forearmed.* What do I mean? Well, given the fear, failure, and false expectations that so often abound, it's worth recognizing that this stuff is rife in enemy territory. As the Apostle Peter reminds us, our enemy, the devil, prowls around like a roaring lion. (1 Peter 5:8) The devil loves this stuff and he does not want a mediated outcome. He wants winners and losers. He wants people leaving under a cloud of having failed or in some cases having been fired. Ultimately the evil one wants festering wounds that can haunt a congregation for generations. A mediator, particularly of church disputes, needs the whole armor of God every minute of the day every day. (Ephesians 6: 10-18)

Understanding Your Authority

We are elders called to tend the flock of God. The work of a Christian leader or elder is to exercise oversight and authority as God would have us exercise it, not lording it over folks but as examples to the flock. Peter makes a long and clear statement regarding tending to the flock:

> So I exhort the elders among you, as a fellow elder and a witness of the sufferings of Christ, as well as a partaker in the glory that is going to be revealed: shepherd the flock of God that is among you, exercising oversight, not under compulsion, but willingly, as God would have you; not for shameful gain, but eagerly; not domineering over those in your charge, but being examples to the flock. And when the chief Shepherd appears, you will receive the unfading crown of glory. Likewise, you who are younger, be subject to the elders. Clothe yourselves, all of you, with humility toward one another, for "God opposes the proud but gives grace to the humble."

> Humble yourselves, therefore, under the mighty hand of God so that at the proper time he may exalt you, casting all your anxieties on him, because he cares for you. Be sober-minded; be watchful. Your adversary the devil prowls around like a roaring lion, seeking someone to devour. Resist him, firm in your faith, knowing that the same kinds of suffering are being experienced by your brotherhood throughout the world. And after you have suffered a little while, the God of all grace, who has called you to his eternal glory in Christ, will himself restore, confirm, strengthen, and establish you. To him be the dominion forever and ever. Amen." (1 Peter 5:1-11 ESV)

It's amazing to me how much authority we can be given. We may not feel like we have much authority, but we do. Especially if you are one who, as a mediator, is coming in from outside and are therefore by virtue of distance alone somehow perceived as an expert.

I believe we need to accept the mantle of authority, but only and always with great humility, trusting both implicitly and explicitly, the Holy Spirit for the light of His truth, His grace, and His righteousness to shine into the darkness.

It is the work of the Holy Spirit to convict us of sin and lead us into all righteousness. May he use us in that work, but let us never think we can do this alone or in our own strength.

B. THE MEDIATOR'S PREPARATION

It is critical that the Christian mediator prepare himself or herself for mediation. Your preparation needs to be prayerful and practical.

Prayerful Preparation

Pray that you will be humble. Consciously put on the armor of God. When you go into a situation that is full of hurt, accusations, half-truths, and misunderstandings, and battle lines have been drawn, you are engaging in spiritual warfare. Paul writes in detail about spiritual preparation in Ephesians:

> Finally, be strong in the Lord and in the strength of his might. Put on the whole armor of God, that you may be able to stand against the schemes of the devil. For we do not wrestle against flesh and blood, but against the rulers, against the authorities, against the cosmic powers over this present darkness, against the spiritual forces of evil in the heavenly places. Therefore take up the whole armor of God, that you may be able to withstand in the evil day, and having done all, to stand firm. Stand therefore, having fastened on the belt of truth, and having put on the breastplate of righteousness, and, as shoes for your feet, having put on the readiness given by the gospel of peace. In all circumstances take up the shield of faith, with which you can extinguish all the flaming darts of the evil one; and take the helmet of salvation, and the sword of the Spirit, which is the word of God, praying at all times in the Spirit, with all prayer and supplication. To that end keep alert with all perseverance, making supplication for all the saints." (Ephesians 6:10-18)

Always begin with prayer for both parties and ask for the Holy Spirit to be a part of the entire process. You might go into a situation feeling more disposed to one side or the other, based upon what you have gleaned from the facts and context ahead of time. You may feel that one version of events seems much more credible than another. You may simply feel more drawn to one person than another. But in order that we might not go in with preconceived ideas or false judgments it is a really good thing to pray for an open mind as you enter into the mediation.

Here are several other issues needing your prayer:

- Pray that each side will come open-handedly.
- Pray that each side will be open to God.
- Pray that where hearts need to be softened or compromises need to be made, that the Holy Spirit would work in each of the people long before you arrive on the scene.

Pray also for the process itself. The best-laid plans may fall apart or be tripped up. Whether it's for good health so all the players can attend, for safety in travel, or whatever issues might torpedo a mediation before it starts, commit those issues to the Lord.

Mobilize intercessors to pray for the mediation, both before and especially during the mediation. Intercessors are often overlooked but they can play a critical role behind the scenes with unceasing prayer support.

I was doing a mediation where honestly it was tough going. By the third day I started my report to the bishop. I had just finished writing, "This mediation failed," when I received a text message from one of my intercessors who had been fasting and praying for the mediation. This individual had a strong sense that there was a special need to focus on humility. As I reflected on that I realized that I myself needed to be humble and not come down with a judgment for one side or the other. Almost immediately I sensed that there might be a way forward and in literally two minutes I jotted down a list of recommendations.

I spoke with each side by phone. They were broadly supportive of the ideas. After I put the phone down I was quite overcome. I fell to my knees and wept. I thanked God for what I believed he had done.

Immediately I phoned the bishop of the diocese and brought him up to speed. He was keen to rearrange his calendar to come to the place as soon as he possibly could.

I believe passionately that God was in this and I'm so grateful to him for that experience.

So often in ministry we get called in and entrusted to do things for which we may not be equipped or prepared to handle. We feel like we haven't got a clue what we're doing, but for a very long time God has been in the business of using ill-equipped and ill-informed people.

Practical Preparation

The second area of preparation concerns what I call the practicalities. I have four simple guidelines to follow:

a) Gather the facts.

b) Read whatever information is available.

c) Digest the information.

d) Summarize the key issues.

I find it is often helpful to create a timeline and map out on paper who's who. Basically, I create a flow chart of who reports to whom in an effort to identify the chain of command, whether formal or informal.

See if you can identify what seem to be the key events that have led to the impasse or breakdown in relationships. The more you are prepared going in, the better equipped you will be to listen and, when appropriate, to respond to things that may come up or be put to you. Your preparation is hugely reassuring to the people you have been sent to serve. If someone is pouring out their heart to you and you ask a clarifying question like, "Are you talking about the letter Bob sent at the end of November?" the person knows you are listening and have some grasp of the background, and that strongly builds trust.

C. First Contact

It's important that the parties know who you are. It may be that the parties already know you but often you will be unknown to the parties. You are simply a name that has been recommended or appointed to serve as mediator.

A letter of introduction is a good way to introduce you. A sample letter of introduction is included in Appendix Two.

With your initial phone call, contact all the parties and briefly explain what mediation is, and what it isn't. Let them know you will follow up with an email. You might also ask if they have any questions about mediation.

D. ABOUT A CONTRACT

The best way to approach the issue of a contract is to review examples. Keep in mind these are only guidelines to consider when writing your own documents. You might consider taking legal advice or asking someone with experience in these matters to review your documents prior to seeking the signature of the parties involved. You will find the following sample documents in Appendix Two:

Sample Letter of Introduction
Sample Letter of Engagement
Sample Mediation Form Requesting Information

E. SETTING THE STAGE

a) Set and confirm or review the dates
b) Assure your clients you will maintain confidentiality.
c) Review the importance of listening
d) Way out of proportion to anything you might do or say, no matter how skilled or clever or experienced you may be, *just listen*. It may sounds ridiculous, but letting people be heard and understood is incredibly powerful.
e) Remember what the Lord requires of you:

> He has told you, O man, what is good;
> and what does the Lord require of you
> but to do justice, and to love kindness,
> and to walk humbly with your God? (Micah 6:8)

Seven

How to Diagnose Without Prejudice

Lessons from a "Turn-Around" Pastor

By The Rev. Canon Phil Ashey

In my vocation as a pastor, church-planter, leader of a missionary society, and as a coach for churches seeking a "turn around," I have experienced conflict. Some would say ministry inevitably involves conflict. I have learned that ministry IS conflict!

Inevitably, church growth, church planting, and church revitalization all involve change. Change, in turn, involves competing values. Sometimes the competition will be between a value that is biblical and one that is not. But in most church contexts the competing values are biblical (such as evangelism/outreach versus hospitality/fellowship) and hence are equally difficult to resolve!

It does no good to the church or the Kingdom to label a biblical value as wrong and take a position against it. All sides need to learn the skills to support Biblical mediation:

- Active listening,
- Reframing of the issues
- Repentance and forgiveness
- Restoration of relationships.

My Own Case Study in Fixed Positions

Some years ago, I was called to pastor an inner-city church. The calling committee assured me that the church wanted to grow by welcoming young families and children from the surrounding neighborhood. The congregation lived in the suburbs away from the inner city, and did not know the people in the neighborhood. Likewise, the people in the neighborhood did not know the congregation and in fact felt unwelcome for a variety of reasons. There were huge differences between the congregants and the people in the neighborhood as well (including differences of race, socio-economic status, and education).

After several months I made an unsettling discovery. The ushers were locking the front doors on Sunday mornings to keep the people from the neighborhood out of the church. The ushers and many of the congregation felt that visitors from the neighborhood would threaten the peacefulness and safety of the church. In the past there had been several thefts at the church by strangers who came into the coatroom or church offices on Sunday mornings while the congregation was worshipping.

But others in the congregation had equally strong convictions that the church needed to welcome the stranger, the widow, and the orphan. For them it was a matter of fulfilling Christ's Great Commission and his Great Commandment to love our neighbors and to make disciples of them in Jesus' name.

In other words, we were facing a conflict with fixed positions: "We have to prevent street people from the neighborhood coming in and stealing our coats and valuables," *versus* "We have to unlock the doors because it's the Gospel thing to do, and we need to reach out to the neighborhood!" To put it in terms of competing values, we had the classic conflict of competing values that run through almost every church: the values of hospitality, welcoming, and evangelizing new people versus the value of having a deep, safe, and transforming community.

Which of these values is wrong? Neither!

The problem is that if we fail to get down to the underlying values, we merely deal with caricatures of each other's positions, so that the positions become increasingly fixed to the point of irreconcilable differences.

Both sides caricatured the other's fixed position. Those who locked the doors caricatured those who wanted them open as unfeeling, uncaring, insensitive to the vulnerable elderly parishioners, dangerously naïve, caring more for the stranger than for people in the church. Those who wanted the doors opened caricatured those who locked them as unfeeling to the neighbor, prejudiced, possibly racist, intransigent, stuck in old ways, and hardhearted toward the least, the last, and the lost. Each side saw the other as not modeling how Jesus would deal with the situation. The big question was how to step back from caricatures and hostility in order to reframe the issues so we could discern the competing values? And with that step, how to proceed to mediate the conflict in a Biblical way?

IDENTIFYING THE PRESENTING PROBLEM

Whether you are a pastor leading a congregation through change or a mediator facing fixed positions, your effectiveness is compromised if you "take sides" and thus become a target yourself. Instead, your job is to identify the type of challenge that presents itself, and then to apply the right kind of skills to address it.

There are certain skills that both pastors and mediators can learn from *The Leadership Triangle*.[37] According to authors Ford and Tucker, theirs is a method of diagnosing a problem without prejudice. It is a lens through which we can ask some helpful questions that almost always lead us to recognize that we are dealing with *change* in the culture of a church (or other organization). Almost always, this change involves competing core beliefs, competing core principles, and/or competing core values, constituting a fixed-position conflict. The authors distinguish and reveal the differences between problems that are Tactical, those that are Strategic, and those that are Transformative, illustrating by labeling each side of a triangle. (They use the words Transformative and Adaptive interchangeably, but I shall stick to Transformative for the sake of clarity.)

When the problem is Tactical, it may be solved relatively easily by bringing knowledge and expertise to bear on it. Leadership or mediation (if mediation is even needed at this point) may be achieved by marshaling expertise, finances, and management to illuminate the situation. There is a focus on the present situation (not the

---

[37] Kevin Ford and Ken Tucker, *The Leadership Triangle* (Peoria, AZ: Intermediate Publishing Group, 2011).

future), and the tone of the problem solving is confident when the problem is Tactical. In other words everyone wants the problem solved, and there is little, if any, conflict evident. The threat faced by the astronauts in the movie *Apollo 13* (not being able to return to Earth safely), and the leadership/mediation brought to bear on that problem by the engineers at Houston Mission Control, are a classic example of diagnosing and successfully addressing a Tactical problem.

When a problem is Strategic it often has to do with direction and focus and involves an evident lack of clarity. Almost always, a Strategic Problem involves not the present but the future, where things need to be planned for and a vision needs to be cast. Strategic Problems can be addressed effectively using (a) internal knowledge of the organization itself, (b) knowledge of the (external) constituency it serves, as well as the broader climate, and (c) an inspirational, innovative synthesis of these factors to offer a visionary direction that everyone can accept.

But when the problem is Transformational it often presents itself as very complex and even resistant to leadership or mediation. This requires a different set of skills than either the Tactical or the Strategic.

Transformational problems involve values, behaviors, and attitudes that are often hidden within the systems and structures of the organization. They may involve the kind of "family systems" and dysfunction that Friedman identifies in his classic work on family process in the *Church and Synagogue in Generation to Generation.*[38]

We often miss the nuances of Transformational problems that surface when Strategic Problems have been addressed, the vision or focus of the organization has become clear, and the people involved realize that this new direction will challenge the status quo.

Transformational Problems arise from perceived threats to the existing culture of the church or organization. The conflicts that arise almost always revolve around competing values such as the kind I described in my inner-city church situation.

Now here comes the thing. If you misdiagnose the problem, say thinking it is Strategic when it is actually Transformational, the application of the wrong skills may actually exacerbate the situation. So I discovered when I first applied a Tactical analysis to the ushers' refusal to unlock the doors on Sunday mornings. I simply reviewed with them the position description and skill set expected of ushers. This approach antagonized the ushers. It was completely contrary to their competing values. Likewise, the Strategic approach of casting a vision of an open-door church was futile because it too was perceived as deaf to the underlying competing values.

As a result, that church experienced cycles of increasing resistance and failure. There was some compliance with authority but no active cooperation. Complaints multiplied

---

[38] Edwin H. Friedman *Generation to Generation: Family process in Church and Synagogue* (New York: Guildford Press, 1985).

around every decision being made. Rounding up the "usual suspects" to solve problems didn't solve the problems. Instead, the conflict and its intensity increased. Fixed positions emerged, leadership itself became the target, and the church soon bogged down in the quicksand of unremitting conflict.

These are precisely the symptoms of Transformational problems that Heifetz describes in *Leadership without Easy Answers* and *The Practice of Adaptive Leadership*.[39] His suggestions for diagnosing problems without prejudice, and how to approach adaptive and transformational problems, have enormous value for both leaders and mediators as they face fixed-position conflicts.

FIRST STEPS TO BE TAKEN

Observing

Get up to the balcony! Most fixed-position conflict can seem like a complex dance when seen from floor level. So we need to step off the floor and "go to the balcony" to observe and record all the relevant data that is out there to be discovered. We must listen actively and attentively to all the parties as we interview them, reflecting back just the facts that we have recorded, as if it were a video without any commentary. We must be sensitive to the patterns and

---

[39] Ronald A. Heifetz *Leadership Without Easy Answers* (Cambridge: Harvard University Press, 1994); and Heifetz, Grashow and Linsky, *The Practice of Adaptive Leadership* (Boston: Harvard Business Press, 2009).

"family systems" that we see in on the floor in the dance of conflict. This is a time to take LOTS of notes.

Interpreting

As Heifetz notes in *The Practice of Adaptive Leadership*, we must listen for "the song beneath the words." We look well beyond what people are saying about the problem. We dig deeper and deeper by asking questions. What else is going on here? What is the "political landscape" and where are its "hidden alliances"? What can we learn from behaviors that seem to be at odds with stated values and loyalties? Are their behaviors (i.e., disconnects) that are at odds with stated values and loyalties?

What underlying values and loyalties seem to be at stake in people's fixed positions? When we offer an interpretation of what is going on, what can we learn from the body language of the people responding? What is behind seemingly disproportionate emotional responses to a proposed interpretation? With all these things in mind, what gives rise to an possible explanation or hypothesis?

As leaders and mediators, we must be willing to articulate what we believe to be the reason or explanation for a problem–all the while not taking personally any anger or pushback that we encounter–for we are not the problem. The problem is rooted in the competing values.

So we must be prepared to ask ourselves, "Is my explanation for what is happening really correct?" Offering an interpretation as tentative or experimental and then watching (and interpreting) the reactions to it can help you gauge how close to the mark you've come. And if you have missed the mark, not to worry, just try again.

Intervening

As Heifetz tells us, "Well-designed interventions provide context and connect your interpretation to the purpose or task on the table." Recall the purpose of Biblical leadership and mediation: restoration of relationships and the transformation of a conflicted church, organization, or group into a functional colony within the Kingdom of God.

Remind both sides of this and have them articulate their common interests. Have them name the losses that are at stake if the conflict continues unchecked. Then identify and name the competing values. Once you have identified the competing values, you are ready for the next steps in mediating the conflict without prejudice.

Futher Steps

Reframe (Redefine) the Problem

To make progress on Transformational problems, a new problem definition must be developed. A new perspective on the problem must be introduced so that people engaged in the conflict can see some possibilities for resolving their differences. Help both parties to understand the conflict from a new perspective that includes the competing values at stake. From a fresh perspective we can direct the focus of problem solving to the "reframing" rather than continued wallowing in the caricatures the parties have painted of each other's fixed positions.

Importantly, leaders and mediators must provide a safe environment for this reframing, through what Heifetz and others describe as the "3-D Process":

- Dialogue:
  Engage all parties by getting their input.
- Discussion:
  Robust discussion of why differing perspectives are important.
- Decision:
  Based on everyone's input go about the task of making informed decisions together.

Regulate the Stress

Heifetz and others describe the process of mediation in terms of a pressure cooker. The leverage for reframing and resolving competing values comes from the pressure that builds up through a process of patiently exposing and facing the disconnects between the parties' fixed positions:

> Adaptive work consists of the learning required to address conflicts in the values people hold, or to diminish the gap between the values people stand for and the reality they face. Adaptive work requires a change in values, beliefs, or behavior. The exposure and orchestration of conflict–internal contradictions–within individuals and constituencies provide the leverage for mobilizing people to learn new ways..." [40]

[40] Heifetz, *Leadership without Easy Answers*, 22 (emphasis added).

This will also require leaders and mediators to protect the voices of those who raise the hard questions and therefore generate distres"people who point to the internal contradictions of the system. These individuals often will have latitude to provoke rethinking that authorities do not have."[41]

Of course, the challenge is to keep this distress within a tolerable range. To use the pressure cooker analogy, the challenge is to keep the heat on without blowing up the vessel!

Return the Work to the Parties

The leader or mediator must return the work to the parties in the conflict because, ultimately, the parties must own the result. This is exactly what happened at Camp David when Israel and Egypt went through twenty-three drafts of the peace accord before they came to the one they could both accept.

The skills needed by a pastor seeking to change the culture of a Church and the mediator facing fixed positions are remarkably similar. Both involve the ability to diagnose a problem without prejudice, to facilitate negotiations at a level of distress people can tolerate, and to help them to focus on a "reframed" problem where competing values can be resolved and then to allow the parties to own a solution they can both live with, no matter how many "drafts" it may require.

[41] Ibid., p.128.

Eight

Mediation Strategies

By Bishop Trevor Walters

There's an apocryphal story about a married couple's first session with an architect. "All we want," they purr sweetly, "is a cozy little house with lots of big rooms."

THE ONE TEXT STRATEGY

Experienced architects when designing a house for a couple employ a certain mediation strategy. They listen to all the requirements of both parties and say, "Well let me try to incorporate what you both want into a first draft that we can improve on." Here we see a neutral third party undertaking to try to harmonize complex and competing values that both parties hold dear.

The One Text mediation technique can save hours of debate and argument. The new house design now becomes the enemy, not the couple's competing dreams. The architect listens carefully to critique and returns with a second draft. This process is repeated until both parties can sign off on the final design.

The final design should represent a synthesis of the "must haves" with the letting go of some "like to haves." The architect creates the hierarchy of what is most important for the spouses, and provides the rationale of why some things will not work. Again, the successive plans become the enemy rather than the spouses' unrealistic expectations, which keeps the pair working together.

The One Text approach is used most frequently where the degree of complexity is high and the competing values very strong. As Phil Ashey noted in the previous chapter, One Text was used by the team of lawyers in the Camp David caucus that led to the signing of the Egyptian/Israeli peace accord in Washington. They kept listening to the two leaders and going away and coming back with drafts encapsulating what had been said. It apparently took twenty-three drafts of One Text before the Prime Minister of Israel and the President of Egypt signed off on the plan.

Here's the good of the One Text method of mediation: If a party says a flat "No" to a draft they will appear uncooperative and resistant to the mediator. But without losing anything they can say things like, "I don't like it very much but maybe it's a starting point." They'll tend to think, "I haven't made any concessions and I can always say 'No' later. Meanwhile, maybe I can move some things in the direction I want." Later on (because they want a mediated solution) the parties can begin to loosen up without capitulating: "I still don't like it very much, but YES it's a little better than the last draft."

The upshot of One Text is that the parties remain engaged with the mediator in the process.

THE JIU-JITSU STRATEGY

The martial art of Jiu-Jitsu involves utilizing the strength and momentum of your opponents to immobilize them.

Counter-intuitively, when you are pushed you pull, and when being pulled you push. You will begin to get the picture if you imagine a larger, powerful person lunging at a smaller, weaker one, who suddenly gets out of the way. With the attacker now somewhat off balance, the weaker can assist the stronger to continue in direction momentum is carrying them, namely to the floor.

Applying the concept to mediation involves avoiding another's strength while flexing with that person's attempt to force a capitulation.

On one occasion more than twenty years ago I had three angry young people in my study, all very intent on nailing me to the wall. I was not in a good place, with my wife dangerously ill at the time. And I was worn out and not coping very well.

The attacking triad's opening gambit was, "Trevor, we think you are an angry person!" They had the look of satisfaction on their faces, believing they had delivered a knockout blow. My reaction wasn't thought out or necessarily a Jiu-Jitsu strategy *per se*, but it had the same effect. I responded, "Yes, you are right, I am an angry person!" (When pushed, I had pulled!) It nearly knocked them over. The conversation ended quickly. What more could they say after that response? Agreeing with my attackers put them off balance, because their lunge was no longer a weapon.

In another example, a mediator of my acquaintance used Jiu-Jitsu when one side found out the other had just backed out the mediation and returned to their original intransigence. People were angrily railing (pushing) at the mediator about backing out being outrageous behavior. Perhaps to their surprise, the mediator readily agreed with them, then he pulled them even further off balance: "You didn't really think there was real money behind the offer, did you?" He had used the aggrieved party's anger against them, in order to get them beyond it to where they could accept the reality of their situation.

PRINCIPLED NEGOTIATION

The classic story told in courses on mediation to illustrate Principled Negotiation is about a man (we'll call him Tom) who crashes his car and then pretty much "crashes" the hapless insurance adjuster. Below is an example of the kind of exchange.

Adjuster:

I am prepared to give you for your car is $4,000!

Tom:

What standard did you use to determine this price? Do you have any idea where I could possibly buy a comparable car for that low price?

Adjuster:

Well, how much are you asking for your old car?

Tom:

I found a used car in the paper for $3,900 plus tax, a total of $4,300!

Adjuster:

I can't go that high. Not to $4,300 I can't!

Tom:

I am not asking for a particular amount but only for fair compensation. Do you agree fair compensation is enough so I can replace my car?

Adjuster:

Okay, I can give you $4,200 for your car. It's the highest I can go under company policy!

Tom:

How does company policy arrive at that number?

Adjuster:

$4,200. Take it or leave it!

Tom:

$4,200 might be fair, I don't know. I understand company policy, but unless you can state why that amount is what I am entitled to, I think I'll be better off in court! Why don't we study the matter and talk again tomorrow.

[THE NEXT DAY]

Adjuster: Here's a classified ad asking $4,000.

Tom: What does it say about mileage?

Adjuster: 105,000

Tom: Mine has only 76,000 miles! How much is indicated in the Blue Book[42] for low mileage?

---

[42] In the United States the *Kelly Blue Book* is used when valuing used cars.

Adjuster:	Well, (thumbing) let me see. $250
Tom:	Assuming the $4,100 as a possible base price, the mileage brings the price to $4,350. Now, what does the Blue Book say about leather seats that are heated?
Adjuster	$200
Tom:	How much more for my 4-wheel drive model?
Adjuster:	$300
Tom:	So let me see, so far we have $4,850, plus tax.

This sort of story plays out every day when negotiators manipulate their "victims" by not giving any basis for their position other than to claim that it is "company policy!"

One is helpless (as was the Adjuster) when he does not have any principles from which to offer a reasonable position. "Take it or leave it" is not a principle.

In our example Tom succeeded because he drew the adjuster out to admit he had no underlying principle for his position. The key thing Tom did was to use the industry standard book for determining the value of a used car.

Try negotiating with a person who pulls things out of the air! "How did you get there?" one asks, searching for any underlying principle that substantiates the other's position. Tom found out how the adjuster got there (completely sans principle), and used it to his advantage.

FINDING OVERLAP IN NEGOTIATION

Overlap extends past a boundary and partly covers something beyond; for example, an awning may overlap the entrance of the building. Or two or more bureaucracies may have overlapping responsibilities for the same thing. Overlap is the near opposite of a gap, which is space between two things. Naming an overlap between the positions of the parties is a good means of shortening the time it takes to reach an agreement. The principle is seen most clearly when the mediation involves money or time.

Suppose Party A's beginning position is that they owe Party B the sum of $10,000. Party B's opening position is that A owes B not $10,000 but $150,000. No overlap in the parties' concerns or objectives is apparent. (The mediator groans, "Maybe this is a gap that can't be closed!") Indeed, maybe the parties aren't ready to negotiate.

When parties are ready to negotiate they are usually mindful of two fixed points: what their "ideal" result is and what may eventually be "tolerable" to them. Christopher Moore describes these as the "target" and the "resistance" points.[43]

This range is also known as the Best Alternative to Negotiated Agreement (BATNA).[44] When there is some kind of an overlap between two parties, if you BATNA their "ideal" and "tolerable" points you will find that an agreement is highly likely. When there is no overlap, as with A and B above, the mediator may be able to stretch the parties' "resistance points" or increase their "tolerance

---

[43] Christopher Moore, *The Mediation Process: Practical Strategies for Resolving Conflict*, 3rd., (San Francisco: Jossey-Bass Publishers, 2004).

[44] Roger Fisher, William Ury, and Bruce Patton, *Getting to Yes*. (New York: Penguin Books) pp. 1–170.

points," if it can be demonstrated that the limits are unrealistic or not in a party's best interest.

It may also be possible to get an overlap by adding tradeoffs to the mix. A church might say to a rector they wish to retire that while they cannot change the settlement amount, he could nonetheless leave early on a month or two "sabbatical" with pay. Or the church might offer to take over his remaining car loan or lease in addition to the lump sum severance that is their upper limit. I have seen these kinds of arrangements work effectively in creating an overlap without moving resistance or tolerance points.

However, a mediator must not seek to pressure either party. The penalty flag is thrown when a mediator takes over the responsibility to solve the problem, and thereby crosses the line of neutrality.

Back to our seemingly intransigent parties A and B with their huge dollar difference. It would be prudent to use "shuttle diplomacy" between them to try to create an overlap that could advance the process. Speaking privately to each, the mediator asks Party A: "What do you think your top dollar settlement figure might be?" Similarly he goes to Party B and says, "Tell me, what is the lowest figure you would accept?" Armed with some answers the mediator now seeks the permission of each party to disclose to the other what the top and bottom amounts actually look like. (This amounts to "reciprocal vulnerability," as the parties have shown their cards at the same time.)

If one or the other still balks, it communicates that they have little interest or ability to move the negotiation. In fact this, in and of itself, is important information that can save the time and frustration of getting nowhere in the mediation.

Let's say that Party A is prepared to move up to $70,000 and Party B is willing to drop their demand as low as $80,000. Now you know that in all probability, a negotiated settlement can be reached somewhere between $70,000 and $80,000. Now, let's see if there could be overlaps in desires or maybe some tradeoffs possible.

Here is another example of finding overlaps, one highly relevant to church life because it involves "music wars." One group wants hymns every Sunday, while another wants praise songs every Sunday. We have just named the "target points" for both groups. Suppose the "tolerance point" of the hymns group is one praise song, no more. Of course, the tolerance point of the other bunch is likely to be the reciprocal, one hymn only.

In this example we have no obvious overlap. What would cause either party to become more tolerant? Clearly here are two fixed positions with only tokenism being offered to the opposing view. To develop an overlap we will need both sides to move from where they are to tolerating some of the music they do not appreciate.

My next step would be to ask each to define what constitutes a hymn and what constitutes a praise song. And what is it about the one or the other that impacts them so negatively?

Now we'll begin to unearth the real underlying principles at play.

The Hymn Party says:

> "It is all the repetition that bothers us so. It sounds like 'How now brown cow, how now brown cow, how now brown cow.'"
>
> "The theology in praise songs is so weak."
>
> "The music is so loud we can't hear the words, much less worship God."
>
> "And it's all so unfamiliar. We can't participate."

The Praise Party says:

> "The words are archaic. They're irrelevant to our generation."
>
> "The music is slow and dirge-like."
>
> "Organ music is foreign to our culture."

Actually, an overlap has appeared, whether the parties realize it or not, but it doesn't yet address a balance of praise songs and hymns offered at Sunday services. Best to demonstrate an overlap on philosophy at this stage, and then to move on to deeper levels of understanding tht will be requited to resolve the matter.

So where is the overlap?

1. Repetition occurs in both hymns and praise music, as *refrain* in hymns and *chorus* in praise music.
2. Both groups value music relevant to their culture.
3. Both groups are in Church to worship God. Hymn singers are open to worship that addresses God as well as naming his attributes. Praise singers are not

opposed to naming God's attributes, but want to worship God as an *I / Thou* expression.

4. Both groups know that music is a means to an end, not the end itself. They agree the end is worship.
5. Both groups are open to learning more about distinguishing sound from weak theology.

Having demonstrated a philosophical overlap you may begin to see some possibilities of a solution. Maybe the initial step is to cut the orange in half in a transitional step, leaving everyone somewhat dissatisfied until, working together over time, a bipartisan committee's good results begin to permeate to the whole parish. Here's what I mean: Maybe for starters the two groups choose the music on alternate Sundays, with each putting it best foot forward. The Hymn Group selects only hymns with winsome music and penetrating words, eminently singable hymns. The Praise Group selects only songs that have stood the test of time and don't call forth theatrics.

Holding young and old together with a common music diet is an almost superhuman challenge. When a church releases a core group to a church plant, the problem is significantly reduced. An important point in terms of their music is that church planters typically have a vision for younger people and are willing to provide music that appeals to the next generation.

THE PROBLEM OF BOOKENDS

Bookends describe a situation where two groups are entrenched with fixed positions on an issue, such as ordination of women to the priesthood. Bookends stop debate. Simply put, the parties will not reach a mediated resolution. At one end is the position that no female shall be ordained to the priesthood (Bookend A). At the other end of the question are dioceses that are committed to the ordination of females (Bookend B). A and B in this case have graciously accepted "dual integrity," respecting the view of those who do not hold their view Having illustrated that Bookends do exist, it should be noted that a mediator may encounter situations that for all worldly appearances seem to be classic Bookends, only to discover (with a little application of skills) that "it isn't necessarily so."

Can an arrangement be found that would be agreeable to both parties? This point may be hard to define if the parties are not at least a little flexible. But doesn't the mere fact they've agreed to mediation telegraph that there may be at least some hope of movement? In such a case the mediator gives it a good try, at least for a while.

SOLUTION VIA QUID PRO QUO

Human nature's default instinct is to avoid giving up something unless there is something gained, known as *quid pro quo* (Latin for, "Something for something"). Quid pro quo is also a negotiating strategy. Consider employees unhappy with their work assignments, with each jealous of the other's good fortune in the tasks assigned to them. The mediator asks both which tasks they would like to surrender, and which of the other's tasks they wish had been assigned to them in the first place. (Of course this illustration assumes the employees and mediator have the power to negotiate work assignments.)

The mediation now moves to the trading phase, where the mediator's task is to help both parties evaluate the equivalency of tasks.

The quid pro quo approach is used extensively in marriage counseling, where household tasks are often readjusted through negotiation. Quid pro quo, or trading, is a very helpful way of maintaining a sense of justice and fairness between parties. Quid pro quo works because both are allowed to negotiate what they will and will not be doing. Indeed, people often have good knowledge of what they are best at doing and what they find challenging or distasteful. Quid pro quo can breed good will where there is none. One agrees to rearrangement knowing that the other must shoulder important responsibilities too. Over time having people do more of what they like to do and less of what they find distasteful breeds good will and good emotional responses.

Nine

The Practice of Mediation

By Bishop Trevor Walters

The practice of mediation requires application of the most effective mediation strategy to each mediation case. As we saw in the last chapter, there are different strategies we can use in mediation. The question of course is which strategy to select for the particular mediation we have agreed to undertake. To help develop some insight in the matter, we shall look in this chapter at three major areas of conflict in which church leaders may find themselves: Failing Parishes, Dismissal of Church Employees, and Parish Conflict.

FAILING PARISHES

The *Situational Leadership Model*[45] can provide useful analysis in mediation, perhaps especially in a failing parish situation where the bishop himself is mediating. I commend it for study by all ACNA mediators. The model,

---

[45] Hersey, P. and Blanchard, K. H. (1977). *Management of Organizational Behavior: Utilizing Human Resources* (3rd ed.) New Jersey/Prentice Hall, ISBN 978-0132617697. Also Hershey, P., Blanchard, K.H. and Johnson, Dewey.E. (2013) *Management of Organizational Behavior – Leading Human Resources* (10th ed.) ISBN 978-0132556408

developed by Paul Hersey and Ken Blanchard, boils down to their being no "best" style of leadership, and that leaders should instead adapt themselves to the "readiness" of the people they are trying to lead. The people's readiness to be led is judged by their *ability* and their *willingness* to accept leadership. Therefore it is the situation itself (defined by the people involved in it) that determines how a leader should go about providing leadership.

Here is my rough-cut summary of the Model (with apologies to the scholar authors who carefully researched and developed it over a many years):

(1) The leader sizes up the people as belonging to one of four categories:

Capable, willing

Capable, unwilling

Unable, confident

Unable, insecure

(2) Based on the people's ability and willingness to be led, the leader chooses a leadership approach best suited to that situation:

Delegating. The leader passes responsibility to group and monitors their progress. (High readiness)

Supporting: Shared decision-making. (Readiness)

Coaching: Two-way communication where the leader is still directing but encouraging people to buy into the process. (Limited readiness)

> *Directing*: One-way communication where the leader tells the group what to do and how to do it. (No readiness)

A mediator who is not their bishop can be brought in to *support* or *coach* people, but of course cannot and should not *delegate* or *direct* (which are never the stuff of mediation anyway). This brings us to the role of the bishop in the case of a failing parish, where he must play the mediator himself and tread lightly until things clarify.

A bishop must be able to exercise his authority although, sadly, I have observed episcopal authority being overplayed at times. As a result, priests and congregations are often frustrated and disempowered by their bishop.

No matter the case at hand (failing parish or something else) a bishop embraces the *twin roles* of bishop and mediator when doing much of his episcopal ministry. Most often he needs to be a master negotiator rather than tell people what to do. Telling is but one of his leadership options, according to the Hersey-Blanchard Quadrant of Telling, Sharing, Giving Away, and Consulting.

Not often, but sometimes, things will be pretty black and white. On one occasion I showed parish leadership a graph of declining offerings and attendance during the previous five years. The leaders were seeking to save the parish but the facts established at the outset brought an audible and collective gasp. The parish had been living (actually dying) in denial. At that moment, it would have been redundant to tell them that as bishop I was closing the parish.

My task was to thank them for their long history of faithfulness, and to empathize how exhausting it must have been for so few of them to have managed so many functions for so long a time. The next step was to recognize that although the parish entity was ended, and some members would be able join another parish, there would remain some who would require continuing ministry. The meeting now turned to how we might go about providing it. Bishops will be pastoral when telling a parish they are closing it, but the episcopal ministry mustn't end there. Not unlike Step 3 in dismissals, some of people will need an amount of aftercare.

Exploring (*spending time*) with the parish leaders in sorting out the reasons the parish is dying can be a catalyst for empowerment and growth. Giving a failing parish some options, albeit limited ones, can be enormously helpful too. In a recent case I spent two hours a month over a six-month period with the leaders of a failing parish. I was able to make clear to them that I understood their situation and developed a good relationship over these months.

Once they knew I was objective, thorough, fair, and had listened carefully to their hopes and dreams, it became possible to share three tough options with them:

a) Close the parish, period.

b) Put a retired clergy in as a chaplain for a period some years to help them to die comfortably.

c) Close the parish and promptly become a church plant, one in which they would be under the leadership of a nearby successful church plant. They would be denied any voice in leadership but would be offered a traditional Book of Common Prayer service on Sunday mornings.

The parish voted to go with option (c) with only one vote against and one abstention. Two years later they had doubled their attendance and were showing healthy signs of life. Recently one of the key former leaders told me how pleased she was with the evident new life as a church plant.

DISMISSAL OF CHURCH EMPLOYEES

The level of anger encountered when dismissing people from church positions is often much higher than is seen in job firings in the secular world. Frequent performance reviews in secular employment result in employees knowing they are likely to lose their positions *unless*. Unlike most other employers, many churches do not hold even annual much less more frequent performance reviews with their employees. Consequently, church leaders may not focus on job-related issues where improvement is needed. Nor is the secular practice of periodically agreeing with employees on their near-term job goals and objectives commonly practiced in churches.

The upshot is that a church employee may be confronted with their poor performance and dismissed "all of a sudden." Of course this results in shock and great anger. Few will ever say, even months or years after being dismissed, "They did the right thing in firing me." Instead, fear and hurt become deep-seated anger that develops into blame and judgment of the former church.

To set the stage to understand this better, let's assume that due diligence has been done and there is solid reason for dismissing the errant or failing church employee. It is clearly in the best interest of the organization that they be fired or replaced. The evidence is irrefutable that the person needs to go. Let's further assume it is likely the situation has gone on far too long, because, after all we are a church, we are loving, patient, and tolerant: we never hurt people! Sound familiar?

On the other hand, Church leaders live with a fear that the fired person can wreak havoc if allowed to stay in the workplace one minute longer once the boom has been lowered. There is great truth to this and action is necessary to avoid collateral damage caused by an angry dismissed staff person. I have even seen church leaders use the corporate practice of taking the keys away and marching the person out the door the moment they've been fired.

So is there a better way to go about handling dismissals in the church? Yes, absolutely.

FIRST OF ALL "PHYSICIAN HEAL THYSELF"

The meaning of the proverb mentioned in Luke 4:23 is that one should attend to one's own faults in preference to pointing out the faults of others. It's the mote in your brother's eye versus the log in yours (Luke 6:41-42) kind of thing. A secular example is the sign above your airline seat reminding you to put on your own oxygen mask before assisting others with theirs.

Why am I saying this? Because when it comes to employee dismissals church leaders have a special problem. Unlike unbiased mediation, where the role of mediator is to first listen to all side of a dispute, church leaders must mediate between their own conflicting roles of Boss and Pastor. For them the starting point is *intrapersonal* and they must first address a conflict within themselves.

If only the Boss in you shows up at the dismissal it is likely there'll be bloodstains on the carpet lasting who knows how long. Relationship is sacrificed for the vision, "We'll be better off without him. He's been the cause of the problem right along. Without him we're free to move forward!"

On the other hand, if only the Pastor in you arrives at the dismissal the issues are unlikely to be addressed directly, while often enough the Pastor in you will give the worker yet another chance on top of the several they've already had. The organization will continue to slowly hemorrhage and for years to come. "Moving on" will have been sacrificed for relationship. In corridors of church power the familiar rationales waft about: "We cannot be seen as unloving." "What would people think if we actually fired him?" "We can carryon with this. It's just a little cross to bear!" How are you going to mediate this false dichotomy? How are you going to deal with the tension between your Boss and Pastor motivations?

CASTING A VISION FOR CHURCH DISMISSALS

We need a vision that holds up the possibility that I, the Boss, could actually be in a deeper pastoral relationship with my ex- team member *after* he or she has been fired.

You are joking, aren't you? No, I am not joking. For at least twenty-five years now I have practiced a 3-Step process of dismissal. My approach pivots on the first rule of mediation: "Always follow the facts." I develop the facts, and I get the facts in front of people. Meanwhile, I have checked all my personal opinions and feelings at the door. Nor, until a decision is made based on the facts, is it time for me to be empathetic.

Step 1. Due Diligence

> I am certain of the facts before confronting the person. I make sure the person has been given warnings and sufficient opportunity to correct or improve their job performance.

Step 2. State the Reality

> I state the reality that their job performance is unacceptable, and I announce the decision that the person *is* fired (not *shall be* fired).

Step 3. Move to the Pastoral

I said at the beginning that one of the differences between secular mediation and a Christian mediation lies in the expectation of an ongoing relationship. Dismissal puts that expectation to the test, doesn't it? What would Jesus do? Clearly he would be loving and, I think, *relational* too.

> I invite the person to come back to see me in a week or two to share their response to being fired. I ask them to think about whether the reasons for their dismissal seem unfair, unjustified, or just plain wrong. I tell them,

> "Come to me and express your anger and pain. I also want to explore options regarding your future. But this deal requires that you must agree not to express your anger to anyone (other than to your spouse) until we have met once more. Under these conditions, do you want to set a time to meet with me?"

In Step 1 and Step 2,.. I am doing what a skillful Boss would do. I have not let my feelings whether of empathy or anger influence my decision. I have kept in mind that the person's own actions and behavior brought this upon them, and that they'll have to live with the consequences.

Still I am very conscious that God has a purpose for their life, and that my task now is to try to help them find or recover it. And I am aware that God can use pain in a person to disciple them and lead them into faithful and fruitful living. (Psalm119: 71)

I Step 3, I am 100% a Pastor working in the expectation of an ongoing relationship with the person. I understand their anger. (Truth be told, they've lost the power of logic for a while at least and resorted to anger as their second line of defense against the more powerful person in the scenario hurting them any further.[46])

---

[46] One time I took over a parish from a wonderful pastor who absolutely hated conflict. Soon enough the leadership team told me that for various reasons there were thirteen (yes, thirteen!) individuals who had to be removed from ministry positions. After these firings, I knew I desperately needed a method of keeping my head and heart working together; hence Dismissal Step 3.

After more than twenty-five years of employing this process, only one person actually rejected me and refused to take up my invitation for a return match where they could unload on me. In that particular case the party was living in an immoral relationship they would not give up. Sadly, they left the church. All the others returned and none failed to strongly express their anger and opinions.

Earlier on, before I was a bishop, I was the one who did the dismissals. Now I am usually in the place of performing Step 3 after one of my clergy has fired the person in Steps 1 and 2, unless the fired person reported to me. No matter except as to whom the dismissed person's anger is chiefly directed, whether Boss or Bishop or both. In any case, whether I did the firing or I represent the boss who did, I can empathize with how it must have felt to be fired. I have all the time and all the patience of a good pastor to hear the person out, but I treat the firing as the *fait accompli* that it is, and I refuse to defend either the boss's or my actions. They are what they are, period. "That was then, this is now," I say if needed.

Helping a fired person to express and manage anger isn't going to change my mind about the decision that was made to fire them, but hopefully it will change their heart.

After 45 minutes or so (my usual experience from sit down to some sort of breakthrough in the conversation), they'll maybe take a deep breath and pause for a moment. I wait. By being pastoral I have already demonstrated I have the strength to face their hostility and engage with them. They are softened, if only a little. The next words are rarely the same, but usually they bear the same sort of a quiet admission, "Well, yes, I know I should have dealt with the situation better."

Because they were not allowed to manipulate me with anger, they have found a new place where they can deal with the consequences of their own behavior. Stated differently, allowing a fired person permission to express anger drains off the power of it. If you can ride out the angry moments, they will likely get down to the pain underling their anger, which is relieved by admitting the shortcomings that led to the firing. The result, hopefully, will be a freshened desire to face up to life's challenges.

I always bear firmly in mind that I am of no use to the person if I allow myself to take their anger personally, or if I become defensive or (God forbid) go on the attack. Likewise, once I have announced the firing I never justify actions taken or the decision. (I will die in the weeds of details, explanations, and justifications should I allow myself even to begin to go there.) That said, the dismissed person does need to process the event, and my pastoral role is to provide time and a place, and chiefly just to listen to them. It is a pleasure if I can responsibly suggest a new role for them in the church, but alas that is seldom the case.

Summary of Church Dismissals

1. Don't Defer Necessary Action

You can do great harm by putting off the dismissal, damaging the organization and, yes, damaging the person too. If a pastor keeps putting off a firing, it will end up making him angry with the worker. Why? Because a pastor, frustrated with the situation, will blame the worker for the lingering lack of any closure. What the "good-hearted" pastor ends up doing is firing the worker out of anger. The very thing the pastor wants to avoid has manifested in spades, and in the firing they annihilate the person, who will have feelings of being banished and long-festering wounds. This is surgery and it must not be delayed or ham-fisted.

The effective pastor will find a way to pastor the dismissed as they feel the load of their failed performance.

2. Don't be a Rescuer.

An over-sensitive (unwisely so) pastor will sometimes seek to rescue people from dealing with the consequences of their own actions. This isn't Biblical burden sharing, it is *enabling* and it is wrong. Paul distinguishes between two kinds of burdens in Galatians 6, using different Greek words for each: *weights* that exceed one's strength and should be shared (verses 1-2), and *loads* that each person is able to and must bear individually (verses 4-5). He teaches that one should lovingly minister to fellow pilgrims traveling the road to sanctification (verses 1-2), while very clearly stating, "But let each one test his own work. For each will have to bear his own load." Each of us must bear his or her own burden while seeking our Savior to warn us of sin and cleanse us.

3. Don't Take False Responsibility

Don't take responsibility for "hurting the person." Let the consequences of their inadequate performance rest on their shoulders and not on yours. You did not do this to them! They did it to themselves by muddling on after needs-to-improve performance reviews and warnings.

So being the boss and declaring an end to something that is not working is not *ipso facto* being a bad pastor at all. In fact, it is being a great pastor, because otherwise the person will continue on course without seeing a way out of an unfulfilling situation. True pasturing is declaring by word and deed that you are going to go with them beyond the former employment. This is about redeployment in the Kingdom versus, "we're glad to be rid of you."

PARISH CONFLICT

Below is a list of common parish conflicts. Perhaps you can add to the list. One can readily see that a local church certainly has quite a menu of possible issues, and that most congregations are experiencing at least some of them at least some of the time. This is rich soil for the trained mediator once an issue has reached loggerheads. The success rate in mediation can be very high in most cases, though it must be acknowledged there can be issues that may never be resolved (see The Problem of Bookends in Chapter 8).

- Triangulation
- Competing Values
- In Reach vs. Out Reach
- Music
- Liturgy
- Churchmanship

- Formal vs. Informal styles
- Clergy Bottlenecks
- Too Many Programs
- Too Many Spectators, Not Enough Players
- Money
- Location
- Premises
- Competing Visions going Forward
- Dictatorial Patriarchs and Matriarchs

A WORD ABOUT MEDIATION IN ACNA

The Bishops of the Anglican Church in North America have developed a high degree of mutual trust and a most hearty collegiality based on a shared history of so many in the Church having sacrificed so much for the truth of the gospel. May it ever be thus. There is further strength in that bishops are quite used to negotiation and problem solving, whether it be among themselves or as concerns their charges. This is a treasure to draw upon when establishing common interests at any of the levels in the church. Godly mediation in ACNA plays forward too, based on a solid record of positive outcomes. Parties may come to mediation within ACNA having a high degree of confidence that the process will indeed bring positive results, whether a conflict is bishop to bishop or clergy and bishop or congregation and clergy.

In any church mediation sufficient time spent together reviewing the importance of our unity is a vital first step in bringing the parties together.

Ten

A Peacemaker's Perspective

By The Rev. Mark Scholander

Mediation is a voluntary process in which an impartial third person assists others who are in conflict, or seeking to reach an agreement, communicate productively, and possibly resolve their differences.

Christian mediation differs from its secular application in that it attempts to address the relational disconnect that created or promoted the disagreement. It is not counseling. Before specific solutions can be agreed to it is important to identify those offenses that broke the trust between the parties. All conflict involves relationships, but Christian mediation emphasizes them. It makes little sense to discuss specific issues if a person's promises cannot be relied on. A former Peacemaker Ministry chaplain coined the expression "Relationship before Issues, except after Trust," or R before I except after T.

An effective mediator is neutral and impartial, two characteristics that pose special challenges to clergy because of their propensity to pastor or counsel. Proverbs 18:17 provides: "In a lawsuit the first to speak seems right, until someone comes forward and cross-examines." It is challenging for someone whose regular parishioner has shared their marital challenge to appear to, or be in reality, truly able to speak to a couple impartially.

In my former Northern Virginia firm Conflict to Peace, the approach to mediation has some distinctive features. First we always use a two-person team and, in family conflict that team is always made up of a trained female and male conciliator. Clients are expected to complete personal questionnaires giving some background to themselves, the other person, and the presenting conflict. We meet with each person in a confidential, two-hour intake session to hear from him or her in an uninterrupted setting their perceptions of why they are in conflict. Following these intakes parties are given some material to read and consider. For Christians, we provide them a copy of *The Peacemaker* and for other clients *Resolving Everyday Conflict* (a less evangelical, simpler text) and accompanying workbooks. At least two weeks following the second intake, both parties are brought back for a three-hour mediation session. The start of the mediation session includes some ground rules that include an admonishment to listen to each other, to give one another charitable presumptions (Philippians 4:8f), to avoid emotional landmines, and to remind them that mediators are not decisions makers.

In mediation, all of the power as to the outcome of a dispute is in the hands of the disputants.

By diverting conflicted people's focus from one another to a mediator, emotions naturally ease. Keep in mind that as parties explain their perceptions and positions to the mediator their "opponent" is listening as well. Oftentimes, mediators ask questions they know the answer to just to have it heard by the other person.

When parties in mediation reach a roadblock, a mediator may caucus with each of them separately. Like the intake, these are private and confidential and allow for the exploration of ideas that might lead to a breakthrough or further exploration as to what motivates the resistance. In a caucus a mediator is free to ask a question that might embarrass the party to answer in a joint session but which may provide vital information.

Like a skilled negotiator, a mediator should be good at creating doubt. As one begins to doubt the strength of their demand, they are more likely to move toward a compromise. Mediators ask tough questions to create doubt or to promote understanding. These questions might include, "What do you desire to accomplish by . . ." or "How do you think they might respond"? The most powerful question a mediator can ask (and that attracts many lawyers, because they are trained to never use it) is "Why?"

Relationship issues, by their very nature, are emotional, including fear, grief, anxiety, and anger. Although this aspect of human interaction can appear in a secular mediation, the Christian mediator should be anticipating the expression of these emotions and relying on the Holy Spirit for discernment as to their source. The ancients had an expression, "Those whom the gods wish to destroy they first make mad." Decisions made in the throes of anger or intense emotions are rarely wise and the mediator's role includes defusing these situations with wisdom, empathy, and compassion. Neurology indicates that once the emotional center, or amygdala, in the human brain is triggered it will temporarily overrule all reason in an act of self-defense.

As parties make progress toward resolution, it is useful to remind them. This not only encourages further discussion it hopefully leads to a tipping point where they realize how much they stand to lose if they don't continue. God instructs his people to build monuments and reminders of his might, acts of grace, and teaching tools for those who follow. Build monuments along the way, if only by listing issues on a whiteboard and (ceremonially) checking them off as they are addressed. If a stumbling block is encountered, consider it like a difficult question on an exam; table it and you may find the answer in a later question.

Christian mediators should remind themselves that they are merely vessels of God's grace and not fonts of all wisdom. Parties should be encouraged to reach their own solutions to build ownership and facilitate future compliance. Oftentimes, very complex matters can be addressed like a Gordian knot, once the Holy Spirit reveals the key offense, or trauma,, which can then be confessed and from which forgiveness can be given. We should also take stock of those life experiences that we bring to the process to be sure we remain neutral and also be willing to share similar stories from our journeys and how they were resolved.

Male big horn rams crash headlong into one another to determine who will become the alpha of the herd. The sound can reverberate for miles in the mountains they inhabit. Eventually one animal, realizing he will not succeed, will expose his neck to his opponent to indicate his resignation. If such a gesture occurs in the midst of a charge, the other animal will go to any length not to mortally wound, even falling off a cliff! A definition of the word reconcile is to cause a person to accept or be resigned to something not desired. Adults make decisions that have consequences. Hopefully the Christian mediator can assist them to make informed decisions but cannot have any ownership in the resolution or impasse in a controversy. It is so not about us!

There are many resources available for those interested in exploring mediation, including Peacemaker Ministries in Spokane, Washington (https://peacemaker.training), the American Arbitration Association (www.adr.com), the Institute for Christian Conciliation (iccpeace.com), and the various state supreme courts, who generally set secular mediators' standards.

Conflict to Peace (conflicttopeace.org) based in Fairfax, Virginia, has further information as well.

About the Authors

The Rev. Canon Phil Ashey

Phil Ashey is President and CEO of the American Anglican Council, an Anglican Mission society devoted to building up Great Commission leaders and Churches everywhere. A lifelong Anglican and "preachers' kid," he has observed and experienced conflict and mediation at every level of the Church. Before his ordination, Phil was a Deputy District Attorney in Orange County, California. He completed his undergraduate degree at Stanford University, his law degree at Loyola Law School (Los Angles), his Master of Divinity at General Theological Seminary (New York), and received his LLM in Canon Law from Cardiff University (Wales).

Canon Ashey is the author of *Anglican Concilliarism – The Church Deciding Together*,[47] showing that Anglican leaders at the global level should organize themselves along the same conclliar lines (i.e., governance by synod) that are so prevalent at all lesser levels of Anglicanism.

Jack Lewis, Esquire

Jack Lewis is Managing Counsel, Litigation for Chevron in Houston, Texas. He received his B.S. from Moravian

---

[47] Phil Ashey *Anglican Cnciliariam –The Church Meeting to Decide Together.* (Newport Beach, Anglican House Media Ministry, Inc., 2016).

College in Bethlehem, Pennsylvania and his Juris Doctorate from Tulane University School of Law in New Orleans. he has practiced law for more than 35 years.

Jack is a member of HopePointe Anglican Church, in The Woodlands, Texas where he is a member of the Compassion Outreach and Prayer Ministry and serves as a catechist. He is a member of the Board of Directors of 25:40 (www.2540.org) ministering to at risk children in rural South Africa to help relieve the devastating impacts of poverty, disease, and violence there.

Lewis is also a volunteer mediator at the Dispute Resolution Center of Montgomery County, Texas.

The Rev. Canon Jonathan Millard

The Rev. Canon Jonathan Millard is a senior priest in the Anglican Diocese of Pittsburgh, serving in ordained and parish ministry for more than 25 years.

Jonathan attended seminary at Wycliffe Hall, Oxford and was ordained a deacon and priest in England. Now an American citizen, he has lived in the United States for more than 20 years, in small rural parishes, in a market town, in a county seat, and for the past fifteen years in the City of Pittsburgh, where he is Rector of Church of the Ascension.

Before ordination, Jonathan was a barrister (trial lawyer) for five years, practicing family and criminal law. He was presiding judge for the Array (Ecclesiastical trial court), overseeing the only case brought before the court in its 125-year history.

Jonathan is a mediator in the Anglican Diocese of Pittsburgh and serves as part-time Canon for Clergy Health.

The Hon. George M. Peagler, Jr.

Judge Peagler earned his AB in History at the University of Georgia and his Juris Doctorate at Walter F. George School of Law, Mercer University in Macon, Georgia.

He is a Member of State Bar of Georgia, Federal Courts of Appeal Fifth and Eleventh Circuits and the United States Supreme Court. After 25 years in the litigation trenches and 16 as a trial judge, George Peagle retired in 2016 as a Superior Court Judge. He recently trained as a mediator and received his license as a Mediator and Arbitrator for the State Bar of Georgia. A long-time member of Saint John's Anglican Church in Americus, Georgia, Judge Peagler is a Member of the Constitution and Canons Committee of Anglican Diocese of the South.

The Rev. Mark Sholander

Mark Sholander is President of Conflict to Peace (formerly Conflict Resolution & Conciliation Services), a non-profit peacemaking organization. He brings with him more than twenty years of dispute resolution experience gained in a management career with the American Arbitration Association (AAA). Mark left the AAA to pursue theological studies at Trinity School for Ministry in Ambridge, Pennsylvania where he earned his Masters of Divinity and was ordained in 2000. As an Anglican priest, he served as an assistant and senior pastor of churches in Florida and Virginia.

Mark was trained in Christian conciliation through Peacemaker Ministries and is certified by the Judicial Council of Virginia as a Circuit Court level court-referred family mediator.

The Rt. Rev. Dr. Trevor Walters

Bishop Trevor Walters is best known as a therapist for his decades of landmark work with burned-out clergy. He holds a Doctor of Ministry degree from the University of Edmonton, where he has served on the Masters of Theology Council.

London born and ordained at Salisbury Cathedral, he was sent to Canada as curate at a parish in Calgary. He served as Rector at St. Matthew's Church in Abbotsford, Canada, Anglican Church of Canada, until resigning in defense of Biblical orthodoxy. He is now Bishop of Western Canada for the Anglican Network in Canada, a part of the Anglican Church in North America.

Bishop Walters is Chair of the Mediating Committee of the Anglican Church in North America, and Circuit Civil Mediator for the Supreme Court of Florida. Most recently he has functioned as a counselor, mediator, preacher, lecturer, and a Bishop in Canada, Cuba, Sudan, the UK, and of the United States. Bishop Trevor is the author of a landmark book *EAS Syndrome – Healing Burnout in Adults Lacking Parental Affirmation.*[48]

---

[48] Trevor Walters *EAS Syndrome – Healing Burnout in Adults Lacking Parental Affirmation.* (Newport Beach, Anglican House Media Ministry, Inc., 2016).

Acknowledgments

To Bishop John Guernsey, who said to me after I had given a lecture on Mediation to some new Bishops, "You really must write this down." I would not have considered such a bold step without his ministry of encouragement.

I am indebted to Canon Phil Ashey who invited me to join him in putting on a course for potential Mediators. This book is incorporated the syllabus of our course.

I am grateful to Dr. Bud Davis, my patient editor, who put in countless volunteer hours to bring this manuscript into the daylight. My thanks to Kathryn Bardolph, who assisted in polishing the work with her extraordinary grammatical talent.

Special thanks to Speed Leas, author of the seminal work on the five levels of conflict, for his generous support of this project.

My heartfelt thanks to Ron Speers, who believed in this project, and committed Anglican House to the task of publishing it.

Finally, behind every good man there is a good woman. I try to be a good man, but Dede is not just a good woman. She is the perfect woman for me. She rejects mediocrity, challenges half-measures and wants the very best for me. She has shared the entire journey of this book, and it is so much better for her mediation.

Appendix One

Speed Leas' Levels of Conflict Model
Levels, Symptoms, Strategies [49]

Level I Problem to Solve

Objective of those involved: Fix the problem

Behaviors: optimistic, collaborative, problem not person focus, rational; language is clear, specific, here and now, adult; real differences over goals, values, needs, plans, information; people understand each other and disagree.

1. Facilitate decision making by collaborative problem solving, or if not possible by negotiation, or if not possible by formal authority action (by voting or leader decision).
2. Methods establish meeting norms, use a facilitator and a disciplined process, brainstorm and prioritize, use communication skills.

---

[49] This is a reworking of Speed Leas's material that he was kind enough to endorse as capturing well his thinking.

Level II Disagreement

Objectives: Self-protection, not getting hurt; solve the problem. Cautious, not hostile; general language to protect people and self no hostile humor, distancing comments; withhold information that might serve the other side or damage your side.

Need is to keep people close enough to work though their differences, not engage in withdrawal or begin to get aggressive.

1. Reduce tension and facilitate people's work together

   Encourage people to "hang in," attend and prepare for meetings; coach people to act, to be assertive, help people fully express their concerns and to listen to the concerns of others; provide ways to build relationships, ways for people to know each other as people, to speak with each other about common interests and needs.

2. Methods include role reversal, expectations clarification, paraphrase and itemized response, brainstorm and prioritize, use facilitator.

3. Establish ground rules get agreement about how we will work on the issue, no threats, identify sources of information, direct sharing of differences, no personal attacks, no withdrawing; norms for meetings.

4. Making decisions, collaborative problem solving, negotiation, formal authority.

Level III Contest

Objective: Win, not yet at level of wanting to hurt the opponent.

Behaviors: Win/Lose dynamics, threatening, difficult, resistance to peace overtures, hanging back waiting for others to show weakness, personal attacks, emotional appeals, limited social contact; language is distorted over generalized, exaggerated, making a case, expecting magic or rapid change, expecting others to read your mind, extreme.

The overall need is to reduce fear and distorted thinking to provide a sense of order.

1. All the strategies mentioned for Level II, as possible.
2. Structure the process and work out a clear process; dates of meetings, time lines, etc. Revise it as needed but work at maintaining a sense of order and direction. There is need for a process that is fair, open, and legal.
3. Use an external consultant
4. Contact between parties to the conflict needs to be carefully managed opportunities for people to express feelings and clarify their interests need to be provided

for each side; at first, this usually needs to be done apart from the other side; when they are ready to work together, then have a carefully facilitated meeting.

5. Decision making should be same sequence as at other levels; however, the more persuasion, compelling and voting the more likely that people will leave the organization.

Level IV Fight/Flight

Objectives: Be hurtful, get rid of the others; being "right"

Behaviors: Factions inflexible, clear lines, strong leaders emerge; language becomes ideological about principles, truth, rights; parties detached, causing each to lose sense of the pain they cause; attempt to enlist outsiders in the cause, parties will not speak with each other, self-righteous, cold.

More tension will require more structure.

1. Use an external mediator. This cannot be someone from the central office.
2. Follow the book. Legal issues may be involved, trust is very low; follow the organization's standards.
3. Communicate through third parties and seek an agreement for third parties to serve as "go-betweens" to carry messages, look for possible areas of agreement,

most likely to be useful when the issue is clearly defined for both parties.

4. Be tougher about the ground rules. Enforce expectations about personal attacks, loaded language; might have a group that monitors agreements and gives feedback to violators.

5. Decision making will likely be by formal authority. Some are likely to leave.

Level V Intractable Situation

Objective: Destroy the others

Behaviors: Attempts to do severe damage to the other's reputation, position, wellbeing; attempts may continue after the parties have been separated.

The conflict is no longer manageable. Outside authority will need to make tough decisions. The parties need to be separated. Some relationships will need to be terminated.

Appendix Two

1. Sample Letter of Introduction

Dear __________,

Greetings in the Name of Our Lord Jesus Christ.

I'm writing to introduce myself at the request of Bishop ___________ who has asked me to serve as a mediator for the people and rector of ________ Anglican Church, __________.

Bishop ________ thought it might be helpful for me to let you know something of my credentials as we enter into this mediation.

• I am the bishop/senior priest/ mediator in the Anglican Diocese of __________ and have been in ordained and parish ministry for some ___ years. I am attending seminary at __________. I've served in __________.

• Before I was ordained I worked as ________________ (include any relevant experience you may have had as an attorney, therapist, in business, etc.).

• Over the years I have been called in to a number of parishes to help resolve internal disputes.

(If you have previous experience in mediation, give some summary of the same.)

• I have also helped settle a dispute between ___________ (add any other mediation experience, if any).

• I am the bishop-designated Mediator for the Anglican Diocese of_______.

I would like to set a date when I can come to visit _________ for X days. I wondered if we could find a mutually convenient time during the week beginning ________ or the week beginning, ___________. During that visit, I would like to meet face to face with various folks and perhaps convene a congregational meeting.

My approach will be, first and foremost, to listen to the various groups involved in this matter and, to that end, I would like to do some of that by phone before coming to _______.

Obviously, we don't know what the outcome of this mediation will be, and I certainly don't make any presumptions or promises as to that outcome. But I think it will be important for all the parties to engage in this mediation in good faith, praying and trusting the Holy

Spirit to guide and direct us all. Full reconciliation and a coming together of the various individuals or groups involved may or may not be possible, though we can and I believe, should pray to that end.

But, in any event, for the sake of the spiritual health of every individual involved, as well as for the congregation, and for the sake of the Gospel witness in _______, I hope and pray that real humility, a willingness to pray, and a spirit of repentance and forgiveness will be manifest by all.

Please be assured of my prayers for you in these coming days,

Sincerely Yours in Christ,

2. Sample Letter of Understanding

Dear ________________________ (the parties),

I write to confirm that I have been appointed by Bishop _________ to serve as the mediator in the matter of the dispute at _______________.

The on-site part of this mediation process is scheduled to take place between date and date in __________. Prior to the in-person meetings I will be having telephone conversations with the parties.

Mediation is an informal, non-adjudicative process. My role, as mediator, is to facilitate effective communication, probe for common underlying interests and understandings, and seek to assist the parties in arriving at outcomes that will be for the good of the individual parties, the local church, and the witness of the wider Church in the world.

I will receive no personal remuneration for this engagement. My travel expenses, including, flight, car rental, accommodation and food, will be paid by ____________together with a payment to Parish/Diocese/Other in compensation for my time away from my parish in the amount of $xxx/day while in ______.

As mediator in this matter I have no authority to make final decisions or rulings regarding any of the parties. This is not an Ecclesiastical Hearing or Court.

It is of the utmost importance that the parties act in good faith. The following are the Good Faith Ground Rules for your guidance:

1. The parties agree to enter this mediation prayerfully.
2. The parties agree prayerfully to consider where they themselves may have been at fault and what words, actions, or attitudes they have spoken or held for which they need to repent and seek forgiveness.
3. The parties agree to take turns speaking and listening.
4. The parties agree to try to understand the other parties' interests and concerns.
5. The parties agree not to engage in negative behaviors and to "[make] every effort to maintain the unity of the Spirit in the bond of peace." (Ephesians 4:3)
6. The parties acknowledge and submit to the pastoral and ecclesiastical authority of Bishop NN.

I have enclosed a Mediation Statement Form, which will provide me with essential background information concerning this dispute. Please return your Mediation Statement Form to me as soon as possible, and no later than _______. Your response should succinctly and fairly portray the dispute.

I look forward to meeting with you. Please let me know if you have any questions or if you require additional information.

Yours in Christ,

Acknowledgement and Agreement:

The parties affirm that they have read, understood, and agree to this Letter of Understanding and Terms of Reference for Mediation:

____

The Rt. Rev. NN   Date

____

The Rev. NN   Date

____

Other Parties

3. Sample Mediation Form Requesting Information

Date:

Re: ______________________________

Please provide the following information to the mediator as soon as possible and no later than ______. This information is for the mediator's use only and will not be disclosed to other parties without your permission. The requested information will assist the mediator in better understanding the dispute and, thereby, assist in effectively preparing for the mediation. The responses to these questions should not exceed three pages in length.

1. Please summarize the facts that led to this dispute/pastoral breakdown.

2. Please describe the issues that you believe need to be resolved for there to be reconciliation and a resolution of this matter.

3. Please identify the interests or needs that would be most important to you and/or the group you represent in a resolution of this matter.

4. Please identify the interests or needs that you believe would be most important to the other parties in a resolution of this matter.

5. Please describe your attempts to reach reconciliation and/or resolution of this matter to date.

6. Please describe obstacles you believe interfere with reconciliation and resolution of this matter.

7. Please describe your position, if not already made clear, as you consider ways forward.

8. Please attach a copy of any letters or documents that you think it will be helpful for me to see in this mediation.

9. Please read the "Speed Leas: Levels of Conflict" page (attached) and give an honest assessment as to what conflict level the situation in ___________ has now reached,
a. The level you think the conflict has reached circle one:

1 2 3 4 5

b. The level you think those on the other side of this conflict would say it has reached, circle one:

1 2 3 4 5

10. Please print the name of the person answering this Request, and have that person sign their response.

Index of Scriptural References

General Index